BETTER HEALTH WITH FOOT REFLEXOLOGY

THE ORIGINAL INGHAM METHOD

**Including
Hand Reflexology**

i

BETTER HEALTH WITH FOOT REFLEXOLOGY

THE ORIGINAL INGHAM METHOD

Including
Hand Reflexology

by
Dwight C. Byers

*Your quest for health will be enhanced
by having read this book.*

INGHAM PUBLISHING, INC. • PUBLISHER
Saint Petersburg • Florida • U.S.A.

ISBN 0-9611804-2-0
Revised Edition, 1990
Seventh Printing, 1995

Published and Distributed Throughout the World by

INGHAM PUBLISHING, INC. • PUBLISHER
Post Office Box 12642
Saint Petersburg, Florida 33733-2642, U.S.A.

Printed in the United States of America

Dedicated to
Eunice D. Ingham Stopfel
(February 24, 1889 to December 10, 1974)
The founder of Foot Reflexology

My aunt and my mentor,
She remains my inspiration.

ACKNOWLEDGEMENTS

The author would like to acknowledge the very valuable help and assistance from those patient souls who provided me with direction and solace as well as rekindling my enthusiasm and determination.

Their dedicated help made this all possible.

To my wife, Nancy who was my chief critic and editor and who set the goals as well as supplying the encouragement to reach them.

To Dick Shannon, professional medical writer who guided my pen over many a rough paragraph into the intricacies of the human body.

To John Bloch, a very patient and talented artist for his many hours of sketching and illustrating.

To Tony Porter of London, England for his invaluable suggestions.

To Ray C. Wunderlich, Jr., M.D. for his professional perusal and suggestions in many technical areas.

To Gary Fleischman, D.P.M., Arthur Pauls, D.O., Jack Vinson, D.O., Charles Merriott, D.C., Dorothea Merriott, D.C., and Paula Merriott, D.C. for their encouragement.

To the office staff of Ingham Publishing and International Institute for their aid, including Betty Nicholson, Gale King and Jo Ann Trimbur.

To my sister Eusebia B. Messenger, R.N. and finally to those two patient and excellent typists, Sally Jo Barlowe and Carrie Lynne Amic.

My gratitude to all of you for a job well done.

A NOTE TO THE READER

This book and its contents and opinions are the result of extensive experience in foot Reflexology and represent the theories of the author who is not a medical doctor. There may be some sections and opinions which are not in conformance to the theories and practice of the medical profession. The author and publisher strongly suggest that self diagnosis not be attempted based on symptoms delineated in this book. The symptoms as described in this book may be indicative of more than one condition within the body.

In any case of illness or even symptoms of a bodily disfunction, it is advisable and essential that a competent medical practitioner be consulted.

It should also be noted here that Reflexology is **not** a panacea . . . it is an adjunctive to medicine and must be regarded as such.

FOREWORD

Foot reflexology stands the test of patient acceptance as a valid means of making one feel good, relaxing, and functioning better than he otherwise would. As such, foot reflexology qualifies as an important adjunct for health care. As is the case with any therapeutic modality, the skill, enthusiasm, and personality of the therapist are important variables in determining the effectiveness of the treatment.

It must be said that foot reflexology has not yet been proven as effective. One could imagine studies in which patients would be assigned to several groups: one group to receive acupuncture of the feet, another acupressure of the feet, another massage of the feet, and a final group to receive Ingham-Byers foot reflexology. Other more sophisticated tests could be fashioned. Such studies might end up showing all methods to be helpful.

For whatever reasons, we do know that patients treated with foot reflexology feel better, function better, and often improve in the biological and psychosocial disorders that lead them to seek help. It is entirely possible that foot reflexology works for reasons other than those usually attributed to this helpful methodology. The laying on of hands does have special significance for most persons. Laying hands on the feet probably elicits greater relaxation than laying hands on any other body area. Therapeutic touch for health has been shown to be a valid help for persons who hurt and there is no reason that touch for health on the feet should be an exception. The special method of foot reflexology developed by Eunice Ingham and followed faithfully by her knowledgeable nephew, Dwight Byers, is impressive in its ability to facilitate healing in the body.

Quite probably, it will eventually be shown that foot reflexology alters energy flow in the body. Hang ups in energy flow are, in all likelihood, removed. Restriction of blood and lymphatic flow to certain regions of the body may be normalized.

The feet are at the extreme end of the body. Farthest from the heart, blood and lymph from the feet must flow uphill against gravity. Movement of these vital liquids is essential. As with any stream, heavy particles will tend to settle out as sediment, especially when the current is not swift. Also, sluggish flow may promote poor oxygenation of tissues and inadequate removal of waste. Sludging of blood may occur, further hindering blood flow. Crystals in tissues may form.

There are 7,200 nerve endings in each foot. Perhaps this fact, more than any other, explains why we feel so much better when our feet are treated. Nerve endings in the feet have extensive interconnections through the spinal cord and brain with all areas of the body. Surely the feet are a gold mine of opportunity to release tension and enhance health. The Ingham-Byers method of foot reflexology deserves wide usage as a valuable adjunct to the medical care of patients in need.

Ray C. Wunderlich Jr., M.D.

Ray C. Wunderlich Jr., M.D.
Preventive Medicine and
Health Promotion
St. Petersburg, Florida
March, 1983

FOREWORD

Good health is so precious that every possible means to achieve this state must be considered and applied. The Science of Reflexology developed as one of these means, by which special, learned techniques locate exactly where disorders occur, and then returns normal function to the respective tissues and organs.

I have been associated with Reflexology for over a decade, and I apply it in my practice for rehabilitation of disabilities. As a Doctor of Podiatric Medicine, I search always for improved methods of treatment for the betterment of my patients. I find in Reflexology relief and elimination of many disorders that otherwise would remain uncorrected. Medication, Surgery, Acupuncture, Biomechanics and Physical Therapy comprise much of my work, yet Reflexology continues to be an essential aide either by itself or with other modes of therapy.

Dwight C. Byers wrote this up-dated volume from years of experience and dedicated research. He offers scientific descriptions and easy-to-follow applications not available in any other book dealing with this subject. Delightful down-to-earth comments and personal explanations create an imagined sense of attending a Reflexology Seminar. Still the same tradition of professional writing standards, found in books by Eunice Ingham, exist here to be enjoyed with educational benefit by people in all fields of health. The book not only covers techniques of working both feet and hands but also, as related to reflexology, it describes anatomy and physiology of body systems, disease processes and referral areas between the upper and lower torso and extremities.

It is my hope that my Medical and Surgical Colleagues will see the proven value of Reflexology as an effective disease-fighting method. For the end result strives to provide wholesome, long life for us all.

Sincerely,

Gary F. Fleischman, D.P.M.

Member of American Podiatry Association
Member of Connecticut Podiatry Association
Member of American Public Health Association
Member of American Academy of Podiatric Acupuncture
Member of United States Congressional Advisory Board
Served two terms as Chairman of The Board of Health,
Milford, Connecticut

FOREWORD

It gives me great pleasure to write this foreword for my friend, Dwight Byers. I first met Dwight during a lecture tour I was making of the U.S.A. in 1976. I, as the founder of Ortho-Bionomy, was introducing my therapy to see if there was an interest for yet another new form of body work.

Whilst in Houston, I took a seminar on Reflexology conducted by Dwight Byers. He taught it with great clarity and understanding of the subject and I was very impressed by his knowledge and experience, coupled with many years of research into the therapy.

I personally feel that Reflexology should be learned by everyone who wants to understand the reflexes of the body. With this training, a person may easily move on and learn other forms of reflex work, such as Ortho-Bionomy and find they learn more rapidly, because the learning of Reflexology (as taught by Mr. Byers) gives a person the necessary touch needed in healing.

The system of Reflexology is safe, yet extremely effective in many cases where other therapies have failed to bring results. I use the technique often in my general practice of Ortho-Bionomy and Osteopathy.

I would remind the reader that however good a book is, it becomes better when the study of it is coupled with practical experience. This is gained in a seminar given by someone who not only fully understands the subject, but who, like Dwight Byers, has the 'knack' of making the good work both educational and interesting.

Reflexology today is growing by leaps and bounds and the teaching of it, due to Mr. Byers and carefully selected assistants, is showing persons in all walks of life that it is possible to help ourselves and our fellow man.

I feel Reflexology is one of the real natural alternatives that can only make any other therapy better by its inclusion into any healing programme.

Dwight Byers is a tireless worker and is a credit to this alternative field of healing. I feel he is doing a great service to mankind in his educational approach to health, not only in the therapeutic line, but in the preventative field as well.

I trust this book will aid those whose interest lies in this field and give my best wishes to you all.

Love and blessings.

Arthur Lincoln Pauls, D.O.
Doctor of Osteopathy and
founder of Ortho-Bionomy
Herts, England

FOREWORD

I have been acquainted with Reflexology since the summer of 1952 when I was a student at Kirksville College of Osteopathic Medicine. Eunice Ingham Stopfel conducted a two week seminar teaching all who were interested the location of the reflexes on each foot and the corresponding areas which are related to other parts of the body. She untiringly demonstrated her ability to work these reflex areas in the feet.

During the next two years I visited several large cities where Mrs. Stopfel was holding seminars and teaching this technique to mostly lay people, some chiropractors and a few physicians. I talked with many people and heard many accounts of people with various forms of ill health who were helped tremendously with frequent Reflexology manipulative therapy.

My own experience with this modality has been very interesting. Many times I have elicited intense reflexes on the feet which correlated to known pathological conditions within the patients body. Many of these people acquired relief from their discomfort after working the reflex area in the feet.

This techique of reflexology should be taught to all professional, and especially non-professional people who have a desire to seek treatment for bodily ailments other than, or even in conjunction with orthodox medical approaches of illness.

I am pleased to recommend this book and the teachings of Dwight C. Byers in the application of Reflexology.

Jack R. Vinson, D.O.
Dallas, Texas

FOREWORD

When we first learned about the book Dwight Byers has written on Reflexology it caused us to reflect on the past association we have had as a family with Fred & Eunice Stopfel and later with the Byers family as they carried on the teaching of Reflexology.

Our first experience with Reflexology began with a course taken in 1959 given by Eunice Ingham Stopfel. The results obtained in this first class were so beneficial to both my family and our patients that my husband and daughter and I attended every class Mrs. Stopfel gave in Arizona.

The benefits received by our patients in the use of Reflexology in our Chiropractic practice has been phenomenal. As Doctors of Chiropractic it has enhanced our work. It has been a great help in many problem cases.

We feel there is total commitment on the part of Dwight Byers to carry on the dedication of his aunt Eunice Ingham Stopfel to further the teachings she began so many years ago.

Best wishes for continued growth in spreading the healthful benefits from Reflexology.

Dr. Dorothea I. Merriott

Dr. Charles E. Merriott

Dr. Paula J. Merriott
Phoenix, Arizona

PREFACE

When faced with the question of "why this book?", I
hesitate to answer for fear that I may not adequately answer
all of the reasons.

But perhaps a few will suffice for the time.

The first, and I feel the most compelling reason is the simple
and rather obvious fact that the time has come to establish
(or should I say "re-establish") those basic tenets put forth
so clearly by my Aunt Eunice Ingham in her books: *Stories
the Feet Can Tell Thru Reflexology*, and *Stories the Feet
Have Told Thru Reflexology*. These books, together with
her seminar teaching and original research, clearly establish
her as the founder of foot Reflexology as it is known today.

For some years, these books remained the basic guideline to
the science of Reflexology. They were a basic history of her
work as she struggled to evolve this most interesting approach to better health. Anyone who has read through
these two books suddenly realizes that Eunice Ingham did
indeed, add the needed dimensions of knowledge and the
impetus in making Reflexology work.

Today, as I read some of the books on the subject, I become
concerned that somewhere along the way, the Original
Eunice Ingham Method of Reflexology has become con-
taminated with mistruths and perhaps just a bit off target.

This statement is based upon my observations as I travel
throughout the world and my reading all of the available information on the subject; there are so-called disciples of
Reflexology whose claims are somewhat spurious and
whose teaching lacks genuine authority. My attention has
been directed to so-called schools of Reflexology . . . they
are neither schools nor do they teach true Reflexology!

I have always held my Aunt's view that Reflexology is a
science. True, it is one in which we do not know *all* the
answers . . . but nevertheless, it is a science that should not
be exploited to the point where reason is abandoned for
pure gain.

This has led me to write this book. I want it to be the **most complete** and **authoritative** reference manual available on the subject of Reflexology.

It has not been an easy task. I have spent much time poring over my Aunt's original writings, correspondence and notes . . . from these, has evolved the second reason for this book.

My second purpose in developing this book is the very same as the one I use in teaching seminars in Reflexology to thousands of students in hundreds of seminars . . . to continue to develop Reflexology as a science by sharing my knowledge of the subject with those who seriously consider the goals of Reflexology to be that of helping their fellow human beings.

This was the basic goal of Eunice Ingham . . . as it remains mine today . . . to help mankind as much as we are able whenever possible and wherever we might be. This goal has been partially reached through our many seminars and the distribution of bulletins from the International Institute of Reflexology. Now, with the publication of this book we are able to communicate on an even greater scale and in far greater depth.

But the message remains the same . . . Reflexology is not a commodity for sale; rather, it is a dedication to a single purpose . . . bringing help and better health to our fellow humans in a natural way.

If you share this dedication and become a Reflexologist . . . let it be your goal, today, tomorrow and for all your tomorrows.

But we would caution you to remember that Reflexology is constantly changing . . . everything is not in this book, nor *any* book. The secret to becoming a successful Reflexologist is continuing education and practice.

Practice doesn't make perfect . . . perfect practice makes perfect . . . continuing updated education makes practice more perfect. And as you progress through the information presented in this book, you will learn of the truth in my favorite adage, "Experience is the Father of All Knowledge."

DWIGHT C. BYERS

CONTENTS

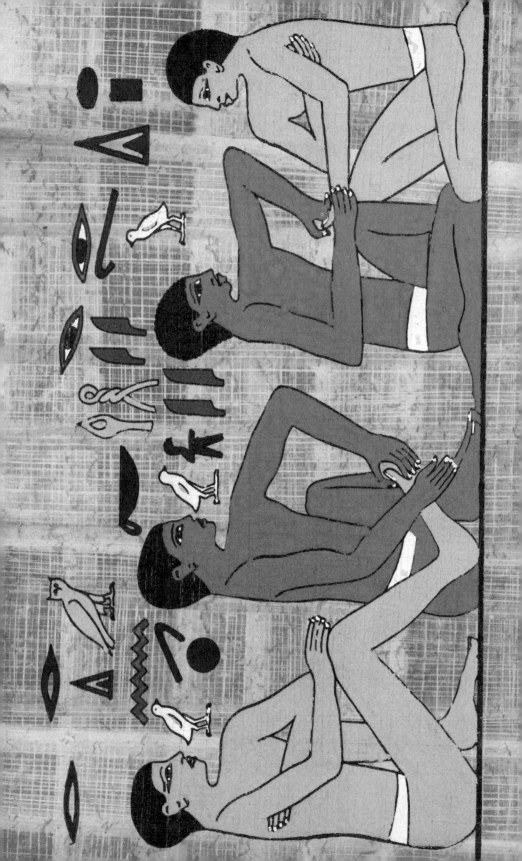

Chapter 1

HISTORY OF REFLEXOLOGY

"Beloved, I wish above all things that thou mayest prosper and be in health, even as thy soul prospereth."

3 John 2

EGYPTIAN REFLEXOLOGY TREATMENT

Early 6th dynasty about 2,330 B.C. wall painting in tomb of Ankhmahor (highest official after the king) at Saqqara, and is known as the physicians tomb. Translation reads "Don't hurt me". The practitioner's reply:—"I shall act so you praise me."

HISTORY

Not being a qualified explorer of antiquity, I must allow those who are far better equipped than myself to study the origins of this science of Reflexology. I will only add this small contribution to their search: Its origins evidently reach back into ancient Egypt as evidenced by inscriptions found in a physician's tomb (*mastaba*) in Egypt. The hieroglyphics and their translation are shown on **page 1.**

Just what relationship Reflexology, as we know it today has with the very ancient art of Oriental Pressure Therapy is still unknown. There would seem to be quite a distinct relationship to the two sciences; my own personal feeling is that it does serve as a link to the ancient art as practiced by the early Egyptians. Then, of course, we read in the Bible of the traditions associated with the feet, that of washing them, etc. Could this be another historical hint?

There are just too many coincidences to gloss over when studying the history of our science today, but once again let me add that I am not a medical historian so I will leave those clues to those who delve into the dim past.

The trip through time to our present age is a somewhat different matter. My initiation into Reflexology came as a youth when I served as one of the *guinea pigs* for my Aunt Eunice Ingham as she was developing the state-of-the-art in this science. But more of those experiences later.

I suppose that anyone who wanted to study the history of modern Reflexology should begin with a Doctor William H. Fitzgerald, among others.

The reason why I chose to begin with this gentleman becomes clear as the result of a search through the faded, yellow newspaper clippings of my Aunt Eunice. One of the clippings is dated April 29, 1934; the headline reads:

MYSTERY OF ZONE THERAPY EXPLAINED

The article tells of a dinner party at which one of the guests was Dr. William H. Fitzgerald, touted as "the discoverer of zone therapy."

In 1917, Dr. Fitzgerald published a most interesting book with the title *Zone Therapy, or Relieving Pain At Home*. In the book, he describes his success with relieving pain through the use of various devices on the hands and fingers.

It so happened that at that fateful dinner was a well-known concert singer who had announced that the upper register tones of her voice had gone flat and the article noted that throat specialists had been unable to discover the cause of this affliction. Dr. Fitzgerald, according to the newspaper article, asked to examine the fingers and toes of the singer. After his examination, he told her that the cause of the loss of her upper tones was a callus on her right great toe. After applying pressure to the corresponding part in the same zone for a few minutes, the patient remarked that the pain in her toe had disappeared. Then, to quote from the article, "whereupon the doctor asked her to try the tones of the upper register. Miraculously, it seemed to us, the singer reached two notes higher than she had ever sung before."

Incredible?

Perhaps to the reporter writing that story, but to one who was under the tutelage of my Aunt Eunice, it was an everyday occurrence.

But what did that dinner party held so many years ago have to do with our current concepts of Reflexology?

Dr. Fitzgerald was a physician at the Boston City Hospital as well as a practicing laryngologist at St. Francis Hospital in Hartford, Connecticut. He had also studied in Vienna, as well as other places in Europe, and was for two years on the staff of the Central London Ears, Nose and Throat Hospital. It was in 1902 while he was head of the Nose and Throat Department that he became acquainted with zone therapy. He worked with the hands by applying pressure to various parts of the fingers in order to relieve pain. It should be noted here that he used a variety of appliances . . . but it *was* quite successful.

The seed was planted; the beginnings of what we know today as Reflexology were fundamentally written in that book. The book itself made no great impact upon the medical world and gathered dust on many a physician's shelf . . . except for one who was intrigued by this theory of zone therapy.

To him, it presented a distinct possibility which ought to be explored. He expressed this thought and wishes to his staff therapist. The seed started to grow.

The physician's name was Dr. Joe Shelby Riley.

And working as a therapist in his office was one Eunice Ingham.

Dr. Riley became interested in the work being done by Dr. Fitzgerald but did not actively pursue it. Eunice Ingham was also interested in zone therapy because of the extensive work she was doing as a therapist. They had discussed the theory many times until the desire to know more about the theory became almost an obsession with Eunice Ingham. She knew that Fitzgerald concentrated mainly on the hands with his theory . . . but, if the hands responded to this treatment . . . there was one other corresponding part of the body which was even more sensitive . . . the foot. After explaining this theory to Dr. Riley and gaining encouragement from him, she began to develop her foot reflexology theory in the early 1930's.

She began probing the feet . . . finding a tender spot and equating it with the anatomy of the body . . . mapping ever so carefully the zones of the feet in relation to the organs of the body.

So then she started working on people's feet using the thumb to press upon certain areas . . . probing and constantly looking for tender spots . . . remembering that Fitzgerald *had* in one section of his book drawn a rudimentary body upon the feet. It is important here to note that Dr. Fitzgerald had recommended using rubber bands, combs, etc, upon the fingers and the hands to deaden the pain for an anesthesia effect. Eunice Ingham did not follow this advice. By constantly probing with her fingers and thumbs, she did manage to locate the tender areas on the feet. One early method with which she experimented was to locate the tender spots and then to tape wads of cotton over these spots and have the person walk upon them. This system over-stimulated the reflexes and caused some reactions. At this point she found it more helpful to use the thumb and fingers to get a therapeutic effect.

My earliest recollection of my Aunt's work was in 1935 when, during the summer, she lived at Conesus Lake, one of the Finger Lakes in Upper New York State. She expanded her research by giving treatments to the residents of this small village. I particularly remember those treatments that year because it was the first time I ever found relief from my annual bouts with asthma and hay fever. She would eagerly practice her theories on my feet while explaining the reflex theory as she worked. I must confess that to a youth who was wheezing and sneezing, theory took second place to the blessed relief she was able to give me. Interestingly enough, it was while treating me she convinced herself that in less serious cases, only a few treatments a week sufficed to help most of her patients.

From this small beginning at Conesus Lake, she was so convinced of the value of these treatments that she determined to write a book, as well as attend all of the health seminars held throughout the country. She did so with the blessings of Dr. Riley who himself was now convinced that there was something beneficial in Foot Reflexology.

In 1938, she compiled all of her experiences and convictions into a book which she entitled *Stories the Feet Can Tell.** This book did more to help her spread the benefits of Reflexology than any other method she knew. She soon found herself on the program at many health seminars. Her sequel, *Stories the Feet Have Told **, was equally as popular.

Among my Aunt's many letters are correspondence with physicians and also medical universities, many asking for more information on her system, others asking her to lecture either at a seminar or in the classroom.

As I have previously mentioned, the initial memories of my Aunt included her working on my feet for asthma and hay

*These books are published and available through Ingham Publishing, Inc.

fever. Later, I assisted her as she held her seminars and there was a certain fascination for me as I watched people avidly intent in learning this new science to ease pain and to aid the body in controlling diseases. It brought back the memories of my own pleasant relief from those afflictions which struck me every summer and I became convinced that there was a great deal yet to be explored in Reflexology.

After serving a two-year term in the Army Medical Corps, I once again resided with my aunt. I was particularly impressed with her new determination to take her findings and results to every part of the country. This determination became a reality through the late 1940's and during the decade of the 1950's. It was during these latter years that she entrusted me with the responsibility of teaching with her at seminars.

But the scope of this activity widened to such an extent that, in 1961, it reached a point when my sister Eusebia Messenger RN, and I found it necessary to assist her on a full time basis. Seven years later the two of us became wholly responsible for continuing her teaching until the mid 1970's when my sister retired. I have continued alone with the development and teaching of the Ingham Method since that time. Of course, all of this work has been accomplished through *the National and the International Institute of Reflexology.*®

In December, 1974, Eunice Ingham passed to her eternal reward at the age of 85 after a life dedicated to aiding mankind and thoroughly convinced that Reflexology could aid in easing suffering. She was on the road with that message until the age of 80.

To protect her teachings as well as her original writings, we formed the *National Institute of Reflexology* and, shortly after, the *International Institute of Reflexology* dedicated to teaching the *Original Ingham Method* throughout the world. Since that time, we have held seminars and named regional directors in all sections of the country and in many parts of the world. Her work and her methods have been copied by some, but the dedication to her original method lives on in the work of our Institute today.

At the present time, her books are still being published and read in seven languages throughout the world.

A fitting tribute to a dedicated woman!

International Institute of Reflexology®
presents
Advanced Ingham Method™ Seminars

- **Theory, Demonstration and Instruction** based on over 55 years of research and teaching are combined in a complete Seminar to give you the best possible instruction in the art of Foot Reflexology.

- These seminars are taught with a combination of multi-media training aids ranging from film graphics to individualized physical application, in order to give you a firm preliminary foundation in Reflexology techniques.

- Most important are our authorized, qualified instructors. We have found there are many individuals attempting to pass themselves off as I.I.R. qualified instructors teaching the Original Ingham Method™. They may have attended our seminars, but that does not compare to the training of our instructors. If you have any questions regarding an instructor, please call the I.I.R. at (813) 343-4811.

> *See reverse side of this card for location nearest you.*

The International Institute of Reflexology®
and
Ingham Publishing
presents
The Original Ingham Method™ of Foot Reflexology

Please send me FREE INFORMATION regarding...

☐ **Books and charts available**   ☐ **Seminars in my area**

NAME _____

ADDRESS _____

CITY _____ STATE _____

POST. CODE _____ COUNTRY _____

Rev. 1/95

Chapter 2

WHAT IS REFLEXOLOGY?

*"For the body does not consist of one
member but of many. If the foot should say,
'Because I am not a hand, I do not belong
to the body,' that would not make it any
less a part of the body. And if the ear should
say, 'Because I am not an eye, I do not
belong to the body,' that would not make it
any less a part of the body. If the whole
body were an eye, where would be the hearing? If the whole body were an ear, where
would be the sense of smell? But as it is, God
arranged the organs in the body, each one
of them, as he chose. If all were a single
organ, where would the body be? As it is,
there are many parts, yet one body. The eye
cannot say to the hand, 'I have no need of
you,' nor again the head to the feet, 'I have
no need of you.' If one member suffers, all
suffer together; if one member is honored, all
rejoice together."*

1 Corinthians 12:14–21, 26 R.S.V.

WHAT IS REFLEXOLOGY?

THE ART OF FINE TUNING

The more I study and lecture on Reflexology, the more I am amazed at this wonderful structure we walk around in. The human body is a delicately balanced machine that is synergetic . . . everything working together for the benefit of all. I sometimes compare it to a racing machine which works best when it is *in tune* . . . each part functioning at its peak . . . all parts working in harmony to make the machine work at optimum capability.

Now, when the human body is working like that, we call this balanced activity *homeostasis*. Don't let the word frighten you, it is from the Greek language and can be translated as *a state of equilibrium, or balance*. I will be using the word here and there throughout this book in reference to our bodily activities.

Perhaps homeostasis can be explained by comparing it to our first example above . . . a racing machine.

Have you ever watched a mechanic fine tune a superb racing machine? He works on each part, constantly adjusting, turning a screw here, twisting a knob there . . . until he is fully satisfied that the machine is in perfect running order so that it will get the maximum response and put out maximum energy. A good mechanic will constantly keep that engine in shape, working even harder when something is slightly amiss. There is a good reason for this . . . he knows that even the slightest component of an engine has to work as well, and as hard, as the largest part. And, if it doesn't . . . then the whole engine is out of tune . . . it will not be working at maximum efficiency.

Now, let's compare the analogy to your own body. As I stated before, your body is a finely tuned wonder. The healthy human body is an amazing machine with everything working in perfect order, the balance being maintained through a system of glands, organs, nerves, chemicals, etc. But let one of these components get out of order, and the effect is felt throughout the entire body system. You are out of *tune*.

And that is the basis for Reflexology.

The principles of Reflexology embody the techniques designed to keep the body's systems operating at peak efficiency . . . or keeping your body *tuned up*.

How?

Well, let's look at my definition of Reflexology.

THE DEFINITION OF FOOT AND HAND REFLEXOLOGY

Reflexology is a science that deals with the principle that there are reflex areas in the feet and hands which correspond to all of the glands, organs and parts of the body. Reflexology is a unique method of using the thumb and fingers on these reflex areas.

Foot and hand Reflexology includes, but is not limited to, use:

(1) to relieve stress and tension.

(2) to improve blood supply and promote the unblocking of nerve impulses.

(3) to help nature achieve homeostasis.

REFLEXOLOGY RELAXES TENSION

Since approximately 75% of today's diseases are attributable to stress and tension, various body systems are affected in different ways and to varying degrees. One person may exhibit cardiovascular problems, another gastrointestinal upset, anorexia, palpitations, sweating, headaches . . . to mention but a few of the myriad of bodily reactions to stress. Often in my seminars I describe tension as a tourniquet around the body's system . . . a tightening that can lead to serious consequences. I will be discussing stress and tension in much more detail later in this book, always emphasizing its debilitating effects.

REFLEXOLOGY IMPROVES NERVE AND BLOOD SUPPLY

In order to keep the body at a normal balance, it is imperative that the blood and nerve supply to every organ and gland be at a maximum. Of course, the organs and glands contribute to the overall well-being of the body . . . each making contributions to maintaining an efficient, fully-operated mechanism, but all receive their *instructions* from the most intricate of all networks, the nerves.

These cord-like structures, comprised of a collection of nerve fibers, convey impulses between a part of the central nervous system and other regions of the body. They are the *wiring system* of the *house* you call your body. As with any complex wiring system, a *short circuit* can mean trouble.

A short circuit is often caused by tension putting pressure on a vital nerve plexus or even a single nerve structure supplying a vital organ.

As tension is eased, pressure on the nerves and vessels is relaxed, thus improving the flow of blood and its oxygen-rich nutrients to all parts of the body.

REFLEXOLOGY HELPS NATURE TO NORMALIZE

Overactive glands or organs can be helped to return to normal. Conversely, if an organ or a gland is underactive, Reflexology can help return it to its normally functioning level. It is important to note here that the normalization action of Reflexology is never one of opposite extreme. In other words, once homeostasis or a normal condition is achieved, it cannot be *unbalanced* by working the area too much. Overworking can cause some minor reactions such as diarrhea or perhaps some nasal mucus being secreted (runny nose). These reactions though are cleansing poisons from the body. Succinctly, Reflexology cannot harm a system, it simply brings it back into balance.

NOTE: Before we continue, let me just insert a word of warning. Unless you are a licensed physician you should never:

- Diagnose: name a disease

- Prescribe: never prescribe anything nor adjust their medication.

- Treat for a specific condition

THE ZONE THEORY

As I have previously mentioned, Reflexology embodies the relationship of the reflexes in the feet to all of the glands and organs in the body. Let's now discuss that relationship. Just how does one small area of the foot affect something like the pituitary gland?

Just what is the *link*?

This is where the ZONE THEORY becomes significantly important to every Reflexologist. To repeat my analogy: the zones are like the wiring in a house, the reflexes travel through the zones similar to electricity through the wires. But please note that this analogy is not to be confused with the nervous system in the body . . . *reflexes* as far as we know today, are **not** nerves.

The link from the feet to the organs and the glands in the body is a series of imaginary longitudinal lines each encompassing a zone.

The word *zone* is used for several significant reasons . . . but first, let's take a closer look at just what constitutes the zone theory.

There are ten (10) lines or *zones*. Easy enough to remember: one for each finger, or, one for each toe.

As the illustration shows, these zones run the entire length of the body . . . from the top of the head to the tips of the toes. (**See Figure 2.1**).

It is extremely important that Reflexologists become *zone oriented* in that they must be thoroughly familiar with the basic zones and the anatomy associated within them.

Let's present another analogy which will serve to give you a better and clearer understanding of the zone theory.

Let's bake a fruit cake in the shape of a gingerbread man. And then fill it with all of those things one generally finds in such a concoction . . . fruits and nuts and bits of spices and whatever else the cook decides to throw in. Now, when our little man is finally done, we are going to take him and make ten slices longitudinally . . . from top to bottom (**See Figure 2.2**). Each of these longitudinal slices represents a

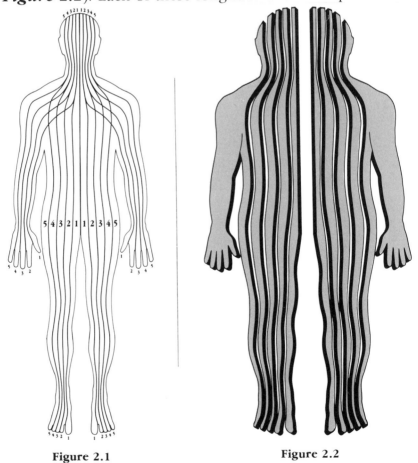

Figure 2.1   Figure 2.2

zone. Everything within that slice (zone) belongs to that zone . . . from head to toe and from front to back.

Got the picture?

Look at the illustration again. Now, take a good look at your own body. Think of your body marked with these ten zones. Start with the small toe, that is a zone. Notice how that zone extends from the small toe right on up to the top of your head. Next, look carefully at the great toe. There are five zones in the great toe since it represents one-half of the head. Now, imagine that you are going to remove one of those longitudinal slices from your own body. Which organs are going to be included within that slice?

To help you answer that question, take a look at the basic anatomy charts (*See Figure 2.3*). Imagine that same zone line running from the toes to the head . . . line 1 to 5 on the left, and corresponding lines 1 to 5 on the right. Become acquainted with drawing those zone lines over that basic anatomy and your task as a Reflexologist is going to be that much easier.

And remember: An organ or a gland found in a specific zone will have its reflex in the corresponding zone of the foot.

Any sensitivity located in a specific area on the foot will signal to you that there could be something abnormal taking place.

The importance of this fact can be made even clearer if you return to the basic anatomy chart and run your zone lines over it again. Notice that by working an area of the foot, you are affecting glands and organs within that zone . . . that *slice* of the gingerbread man.

It should become evident then, that by working the entire foot, you are affecting the entire side of the body; the right foot representing the right half of the body, the left foot representing the left half of the body. And while we are on that subject, it is important to remember another significant aspect of Reflexology: an abnormality in **any** part of the zone **may** affect anything within that zone.

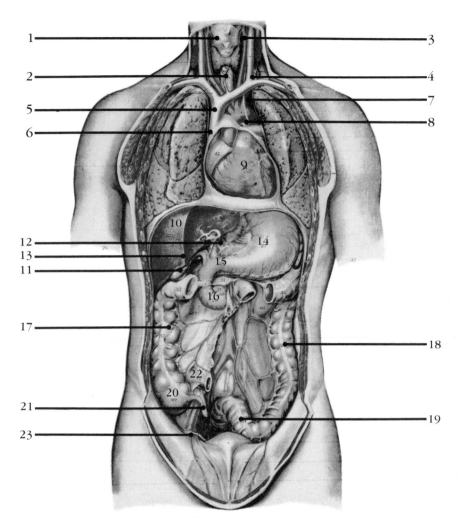

Figure 2.3

1. Thyroid cartilage
   (*Cartilago thyreoidea*)
2. Windpipe (*Trachea*)
3. Left common carotid
   (*A. carotis communis sinistra*)
4. Thoracic duct (*Ductus thoracicus*)
5. Superior cava (*V. cava superior*)
6. Pericardium (*Pericardium*)
7. Phrenic (*N. phrenicus*)
8. Vagus (*N. vagus*)
9. Heart (*Cor*)
10. Liver (*Hepar*)
11. Gall bladder (*Vessica fellea*)
12. Hepatic artery, portal vein,

hepatic duct (*A. hepatica propria,
V. portae, ductus hepaticus*)
13. Foramen of Winslow
    (*Foramen epiploicum*)
14. Stomach (*Ventriculus*)
15. Pylorus (*Pylorus*)
16. Duodenum (*Duodenum*)
17. Ascending colon (*Colon ascendens*)
18. Descending colon (*Colon descendens*)
19. Sigmoid (*Colon sigmoideum*)
20. Blind intestine (*Caecum*)
21. Appendix (*Processus vermiformis*)
22. Ileum (*Ileum*)
23. Spermatic duct (*Ductus deferens*)

16

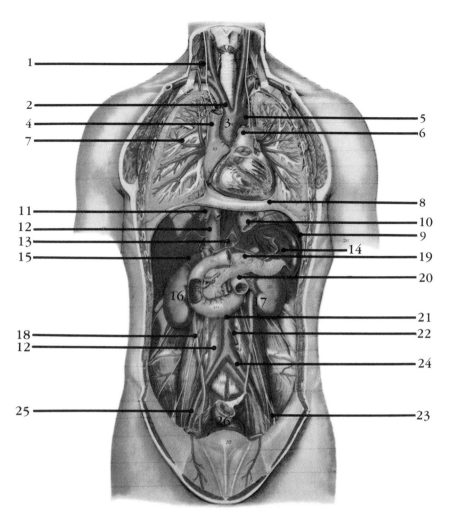

Figure 2.3

1. Vertebral (*A. vertebralis*)
2. Brachiocephalic (*A. brachiocephalica*)
3. Aortic arch (*Arcus aortae*)
4. Superior cava (*V. cava superior*)
5. Left vagus (*N. vagus sinister*)
6. Pulmonary (*A. pulmonalis*)
7. Pulmonary vessels and bronchii (*Vasa pulmonalia et bronchii*
8. Pleura (*Pleura*)
9. Diaphragm (*Diaphragma*)
10. Cardiac end of stomach (*Cardia*)
11. Hepatic veins (*Vv. hepaticae*)
12. Inferior cava (*V. cava inferior*)
13. Celiac (*Truncus coeliacus*
14. Spleen and splenic vessels

(*Lien et vasa lienalia*)
15. Right suprarenal gland (*Glandula suprarenalis dextra*)
16. Right kidney (*Ren dexter*)
17. Left kidney (*Ren sinister*)
18. Ureter (*Ureter*)
19. Pancreas (*Pancreas*)
20. Duodenojejunal flexure (*Flexura duodenojejunalis*)
21. Abdominal aorta (*Aorta abdominalis*)
22. Inferior mesenteric (*A. mesenterica inferior*)
23. Femoral nerve (*N. femoralis*)
24. Common iliac (*A. et V. iliaca communis*)
25. External iliac (*A. et V. iliaca external*)
26. Rectum (*Rectum*)

Anatomical Charts Used By Permission NYSTROM, Division of Carnation

17

In order to aid you in visualizing the significant relationship between the feet and the entire body in perspective, carefully study **Figure 2.4**. Note the similarities of the feet to the entire body.

To become acquainted with some standard reference terms we are going to be using in this book, look down at your own feet as you stand on them.

Take a good look because we will be defining the inside area (medial) as the great toe side . . . and the outside area (lateral) as the small toe side (**See Figure 2.6**).

You are standing on the **bottom** of your feet, and as you look down, you are looking at the **top** of your feet. As you look at your toes, you can bend down and touch the **tips** of the toes. The **back** of the foot is the heel.

Remembering these reference terms is as easy as standing on your own two feet.

18

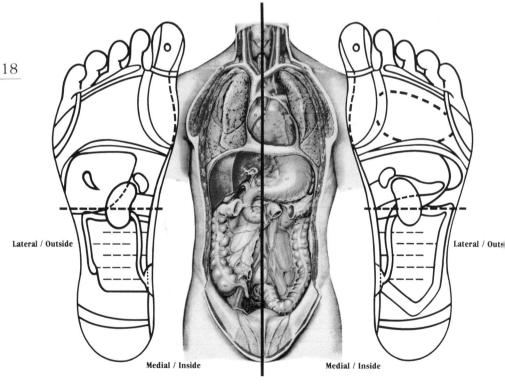

Lateral / Outside   Lateral / Outs

Medial / Inside   Medial / Inside

Figure 2.4

Anatomical Charts Used By Permission NYSTROM, Division of Carnation

And, while we are talking about toes, remember that the great toe contains **all five zones** of the head. That great toe is your general orientation to the head area.

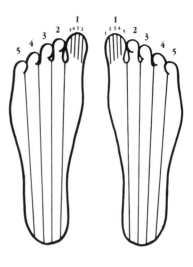

But, this is not to say that the other toes are unimportant; indeed, they are invaluable for **fine tuning** those zones of the head applicable to each toe (**See Figure 2.5**). Each toe, of course, delineating its own specific head and neck region.

Figure 2.5

While we are becoming oriented to the feet/body relationship there is something which we have not as yet discussed. There is an aspect of Reflexology with which everyone should become thoroughly familiar: **Body Relation Guide Lines.**

There are guidelines running either horizontally across the foot or vertically up and down the foot. These are a natural

phenomenon since they represent the all important *plexus* areas and are areas within the body where constant multiple activities are happening; where nerves, important organs and glands are located.

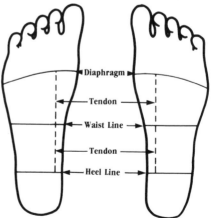

There are four major guidelines with which you should become familiar: (**See Figure 2.6**).

- The Diaphragm/Solar Plexus Line

- The Waist Line

- The Heel Line

- The Tendon which runs longitudinally down the foot.

These guidelines are important landmarks which we will be discussing later. Another landmark with which you should become familiar includes the metatarsal or *ball* of the foot.

Meanwhile, back to our illustration. As you take a good look, one important thing to remember is our analogy of the zone *slice*. The zone areas of the feet are no different. Remember, you are looking at the two feet as if you were looking at our gingerbread man. **The zones go all the way through the feet**. If you can visualize the human body superimposed on the bottom of the feet, you are on your way to understanding the science of Reflexology.

Let's continue with that visualization.

I have already discussed the head as represented by the great toe and the smaller toes. Now, let's look at another of the more important areas of the human body and, incidentally, one which causes more trouble . . . the spine. We will be discussing the spine in another section of this book; right now, we are locating the spinal zone. (Zone One)

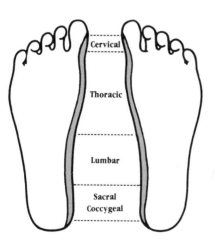

Figure 2.7

The spine, of course, helps to hold the head, therefore, it will be the center or dividing line of the body. But, what about the fact that the right foot represents the right half of the body while the left foot represents the left half?

The answer to that can be seen in *Figure 2.7*. Note that each foot has a spinal reflex area and it is located along the inside edge of each foot.

Anatomically, of course, the shoulder area is beneath the head and neck, consequently the very base of the toes would represent the reflex to some of the shoulder muscles.

One of the more important guidelines runs laterally across the body, and so it is reflected in a lateral line across the feet. This line is termed the diaphragm/solar plexus. The solar plexus is somewhat like a *nerve switchboard* which makes all kinds of connections to various parts of the body . . . a good reason to become thoroughly familiar with this reflex area.

The solar plexus is located in the body just at the base of the body's breastbone or *sternum*. Immediately below that is a large muscular band, shaped like the top of an opened umbrella. This band, the diaphragm, separates the interior body cavity. If we were to take a closer look at this area, we would see the liver, the stomach and also the gathering or *crossing* (plexus) of many important nerves.

The diaphragm/solar plexus area on the feet is just below the metatarsal or ball on each foot. When the toes are flexed back, the foot looks like it is *sticking its chest out* . . . right below that *chest* is the line you are looking for. The chest area is usually easy to find since, in most persons, the area is delineated by a darker color.

21

Now, let's take a look at the second guideline . . . the waist line, another lateral line. This one is a cinch!

If you run your fingers down the outside of the foot, about halfway down, your fingers will stumble across a *high spot*. This high spot, or protuberance, is caused by the fifth metatarsal bone. When you locate the high spot and draw a lateral line across each foot, you have the waist line. A convenient place to divide the body into halves, as well as remembering those organs and glands within each area, is the waist line . . . a dividing *belt line* that makes it easier to orient the location of various organs and glands.

Another important guideline which nature easily points out for you is the heel line. This guideline is found at the beginning of the heel where there is a noticeable color and texture change. This is one of the areas of the foot where the thick, callused skin often makes working it so difficult that special techniques are required. But that is not to detract from the fact that it is a very important area to the Reflexologist, since it is the reflex area for the lower back, the sigmoid colon and associative nerves.

The final important guideline is a tendon. This guideline is located between the great toe and the second toe and is found by flexing the toes back. This action causes the longitudinal tendon on the bottom of the foot to become more pronounced. It is easily located by gently running the thumb or finger over the sole of the foot . . . the cord-like tendon will feel like a taut band. If pushing on the band causes the great toe to *nod its head* you have found the tendon.

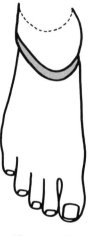

Figure 2.8

For clarity, why not take another look at the *anatomy chart*, just in order to become familiar with these main divisions and the basic glands and organs within each division and then visualize them on the feet.

While you are studying the chart, take a closer look at the groin area. This curved area has special significance when we locate it on the feet since it rounds out to include the ankle (*See Figure 2.8*). The groin area is found where the leg is joined to the body; the groin reflex is located where the foot is joined to the ankle.

ORGANS . . . THE INSIDE STORY

Like a suitcase packed with the necessities for travel, the body is also packed with vital organs and glands in somewhat the same manner. Everything packed on top of everything else.

Once again, a glance at our anatomy chart will confirm this fact. As a means of orienting yourself as to just what foot reflex points cover which organs, start at the midline of the body, the spine. Now, you have a reference point for each foot. Then use the waist line for your horizontal or lateral marker. The most important body organs are located in four distinct quadrants. Now, transfer that picture to the feet keeping one important fact in mind: some of those organs will extend over into another quadrant. So you must work both reflex areas to be sure of covering the entire organ. Want an example? Study the heart. See how it extends over the midline area? What zones would you work to completely cover the heart area?

Once again . . . remember that the feet are a *reflection* of the body with all its glands, nerves, and organs having distinct locations on the feet. Being sure that you are thoroughly familiar with this concept of location, makes the zone theory so much easier.

REFERRAL AREAS

The referral areas are an interesting and extremely useful adjunct to Reflexology. They allow you to *refer* one area of the body to an alternate area, i.e. arm to leg, leg to arm, etc.

Succinctly, the right and left hand are referral areas for the right and left foot. To fully grasp this concept study **Figures 2.9, 2.10**. Note that the palm of the hand is facing

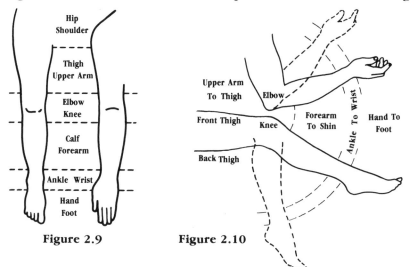

Figure 2.9   Figure 2.10

forward (supine). So this will make the arm bend in the opposite direction from the leg. This will orient you to the anatomical relationships.

- The palm of the hand same as the bottom of the foot

- The inner forearm same as the calf of the leg

- The bony part of the forearm same as the shin bone

- The elbow same as the kneecap

- The front of the elbow same as the back of the knee

- The front of the upper arm same as the back of the thigh

- The back of the upper arm same as the front of the thigh

Also, note the relation of the thumb to the great toe . . . the thumb being opposite position to the great toe.

The basic reason we call these areas *referrals* is simply because of the anatomical relationship existing between them.

For instance, it is quite easy to see the similarity of the ankle to the wrist if we were like other animals and walked on *all fours*. The articulated movement of the ankle would correspond to that of the wrist for motion.

Now, suppose there were a misstep and an ankle became badly sprained. As a Reflexologist, we would know that pressure would soon build up in the area of the sprain unless immediately relieved. Naturally, the ankle is too injured to touch, much less work, so we would work on the wrist . . . for it is anatomically related to the ankle . . . a logical choice to prevent soreness, swelling or other possible complications.

To repeat, a referral area is an anatomically related area

which can be worked instead of, or in addition to, the afflicted area. This is true of **all** referral areas.

One way to remember: when thinking of the ankle, refer to the wrist; when thinking of the elbow, refer to the knee, etc. Your client can be taught to use the referral areas and also how to work on their hands between ensuing sessions. This exercise will reinforce your own efforts.

And why is all of this so significant?

For the simple reason that if you can't work an area on the foot, you can work the corresponding area on the hand, or the elbow, etc. When there is a severe injury, say a broken leg, you then simply select the corresponding area on the arm and work that area in order to help the circulation to the injured area and ultimately hasten the healing process. The basic reason the Reflexologist uses the foot is simply because it is one of the most pampered and protected areas of the body and, being so, is one of the most sensitive to touch. Also, the foot's resemblance to the body's outline makes it easy to visualize the body on the foot.

HELPER AREAS

Helper areas are additional areas worked to aid the specific area of congestion. They are the *reinforcement* you send to aid the specific area.

For instance: a headache. You would naturally work the great toe which represents the head. To help that area, we would also work the neck (7th cervical) and coccyx reflexes as this may be the area causing the headache. A headache is usually telling us that there is something wrong somewhere in the body.

Helper areas are just that . . . they are areas which, when worked, help in relieving tension or congestion associated with the afflicted area. They are reflexes that may have a **direct effect** on the **afflicted area** and are the *reinforcements* needed to make sure you reach the desired results. You are sending **help** to the afflicted area.

Chapter 3

COMMON TERMS DEFINED

"Nature does nothing in vain"

Aristotle

COMMON TERMS DEFINED

BASE OF TOES OR ROOT OF TOES

The base of the toe is found where the toe is joined onto the foot.

CRISS-CROSS MOTION

The Criss-Cross motion is obtained by working an area in several directions, first with one hand and then with the alternate hand. Usually, you will be working on an angle across the foot from the inside to the outside and then from the outside to the inside. The reason for working in this manner is to be sure you cover the whole area thoroughly. Sometimes there will be more sensitivity from one direction than from another.

CRYSTAL DEPOSITS

Crystal deposits are found in the feet when you are working some of the reflexes, i.e., the neck and shoulder reflexes. They will feel like little grains of salt under your fingers or thumbs. You will have to develop some sensitivity with your fingers in order to recognize them. Crystal deposits are not found in all areas of the foot.

CUBOID NOTCH

The Cuboid Notch is found as you run your thumb or finger down the outside of the foot until you reach the low spot. This soft, hollow area below the waistline of the foot will be the cuboid notch.

DIAPHRAGM

The Diaphragm is a thin muscle forming the floor of the chest at the base of the lungs and the roof of the abdominal cavity. The guideline to the diaphragm will be found at the base of the metatarsals where the foot color and texture changes.

HEEL LINE

The Heel Line is found at the end of the soft arch area where the heel starts. The heel itself is darker in color and of a heavier texture. The line is where these two areas meet.

HIGH SPOT OF THE ANKLE BONE

The High Spot of the Ankle Bone will be found on either the inside or outside of the ankle at the highest point of the rounded protuberance.

HOOK-IN AND BACK-UP

We use the Hook-In, Back-up technique when we have an area that needs to be pinpointed such as the pituitary, ileocecal valve, and the sigmoid flexure reflexes. This is where we lay the inside corner of the thumb on the specific reflex and, instead of walking the thumb, we push in and pull the thumb back toward our hand. This is a steady motion where the thumb is *planted* with pressure and moves slightly back towards your hand.

INSIDE OF THE FOOT

The Inside of the Foot will be defined as the great toe side or medial side of the foot.

LEVERAGE

Leverage is obtained by the use of the fingers in opposition to the working thumb or when you are working with the fingers the leverage will be made with the thumb in opposition to the fingers. The leverage gives the thumb or finger the strength and endurance for a smooth contact.

OUTSIDE OF THE FOOT

The Outside of the Foot will be defined as the little toe side or lateral side of the foot.

PIN POINTING TECHNIQUE

The *Pin Pointing* technique is used when we are working a very small and exact reflex area, such as the pituitary or the sigmoid flexure. These are areas that have to be contacted with great accuracy or you will miss them all together.

PULLING THE PADDING DOWN

Pulling the Padding Down is only used for working the eye and ear reflexes. The padding is actually the metatarsal area of the foot. You place the thumb of your holding hand on the padding with your fingers on the top of the foot below the toes and draw the thumb down toward the heel. This move opens up the soft tissue underneath the toes so you are able to work on the ridge formed at the base of the toes.

RELAXING TECHNIQUES

These are special techniques that feel very good and are designed to aid in relaxation. The techniques are also used in working the relative reflex area to help improve the circulation.

ROTATION

Rotation is an oval motion we use with our holding hand when we are performing our relaxation techniques. The rotation is done in both directions. These rotations are used to loosen up an area and they provide a soothing, relaxing feeling. A good rotation will also help to loosen up the muscles and tendons in the back of the leg.

7TH CERVICAL

The 7th Cervical reflex is found at the base of the great toe on the inside edge where the great toe is joined onto the foot. On the body, the 7th cervical is found on the back of the neck where the spine protrudes at the base of the neck.

SOLAR PLEXUS

The Solar Plexus is also known as our *abdominal brain* because it contains so many nerves and nerve networks. It is located at the end of the sternum and in the diaphragm. It is part of the nervous system and it relays its messages through the diaphragm. On the foot, the Solar Plexus is located on the diaphragm line between the great toe and the second toe.

TENDER SPOTS

Tender spots are reflex areas that feel tight or grainy under your thumb and may provide the client with some discomfort when pressure is applied to this area. You can sometimes tell when you have reached a tender spot as the person tenses up or winces. This is the reason we always watch the face of the client upon whom we are working.

TENDON

The Tendon is found on the bottom of the foot when you flex the great toe back. The longitudinal tendon (*between the diaphragm guideline and the heel guideline*) will protrude and feel like a taut band.

WAIST LINE

The Waist Line is found by locating the high spot on the outside of the foot about halfway down. This high spot is the protrusion of the fifth metatarsal bone. After finding this high spot, draw an imaginary lateral line across the foot; this will be the waist guideline.

WALKING THE RIDGE

Walking the Ridge is used when working the eye and ear reflexes. After you have pulled the metatarsal padding down, the soft tissue under the toes will form this ridge.

This is the area that the thumb will be working and it is the only time you will ever use the outside (lateral) edge of your thumb. The outside edge of the thumb will be used in a downward motion as it is walked across this base.

Chapter 4

TECHNIQUES

"And let the beauty of the Lord our God be upon us; and establish thou the work of our hands upon us . . ."

Psalms 90:17

TECHNIQUES

INTRODUCTION

The Original Ingham Method was pioneered, researched and developed in the early 1930's by the late Eunice Ingham and is the leading method of Reflexology in use today throughout the world. The technique used when giving a Reflexology treatment can not exactly be compared to any other form of contact therapy. It is the difference that makes it so unique. The explanations and diagrams set up here should be diligently studied and adhered to remembering that *perfect practice makes perfect.* Without this perfect practice, the all important sensitivity of touch will not be achieved.

As an orthodox reflexologist, you will use no implements, oils or creams as you work the feet; rather, you develop a keen sense of feel using the tactile senses of the fingers and the thumb. Corn starch or baby powder is permissible if your hands or the client's feet are damp.

You can read and study, but practical learning is a **must** to achieve the best results. The very reason that the *International Institute of Reflexology* Seminars are designed: to bring this practical training to you for *hands-on* learning.

Another thing you will learn is to always keep the finger nails trimmed to where they cannot scratch or dig into the foot.

And while on the subject of practical applications, I have found that a recliner-type chair provides the best working arrangement for your client. For you, as you work the feet, I suggest a secretarial-type chair since the height is adjustable and the wheels on the chair allow you to move more easily into various working positions.

BASIC TECHNIQUES

Through the use of four basic working techniques, the Reflexologist develops an efficient sensitivity and the ability to conserve energy by using less effort in working the reflex areas. A good Reflexologist learns through his sense of feel, as well as a developed sense of observation, both of which are fundamental to this science.

In order to accomplish all of this, we will be discussing the four basic techniques:

- The basic thumb technique.

- The finger technique.

- The thumb *hook-in and back-up* technique.

- The *reflex rotation* technique.

We are going to be discussing each one of these techniques and their application as we go from the basic to the well-defined *pinpoint* technology. But first, we are going to consider the fact that no matter how well we develop these working techniques, we can not really accomplish our goal unless we learn one other basic and elementary tenet of Reflexology . . . the proper holding of the feet. There are many reasons for the various configurations for holding the feet properly, and they will be discussed as we develop each of the techniques. The procedures being described here are all depicted as I would work on a client . . . their right foot will be on my left, and vice versa.

35

Since Reflexology works with both feet and since the reflex areas can be worked with both hands, the hand which will be working the reflex areas will now be termed the *working* hand. The other hand which naturally works as an adjunctive to the working hand, will be called the *holding* hand.

Each of the techniques we will be describing has its own holding as well as working techniques, so it is important for the trained Reflexologist not only to develop the four working techniques, but also to become familiar with the adjunctive holding techniques which allow them to acquire a cooperative effect and thus a more successful application of Reflexology. I would like you to remember it this way: to successfully work the feet, we need teamwork with the hands.

BASIC HOLDING TECHNIQUE

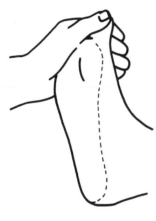

Figure 4.1

The heel of your holding hand will be placed against the metatarsals of the foot with the fingers lightly wrapped over the toes and the thumb pressed lightly against either the great toe or the small toe, depending on which hand you are using. This gives you control over the foot and allows you to push the foot back or to bring it forward. This specific hold will be used for the majority of the techniques utilized on the bottom of the foot. (*See Figure 4.1*).

THE BASIC THUMB TECHNIQUE

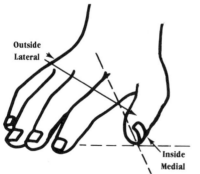

Outside
Lateral

Inside
Medial

Figure 4.2

For the beginning Reflexologist, the thumb technique is a very basic one and can be best demonstrated by placing your hand palm down on a table (*See Figure 4.2*). You will notice the natural position of your hand on the table and particularly the angle of the thumb where it meets the table, this is going to be the **working area** of the thumb. The inside (medial) edge of the thumb makes contact with the table. This is the part of the thumb that you should be using . . . **inside (medial) corresponds to the *inside of the foot* . . . outside (lateral) corresponds to the *outside of the foot.***

You will notice that your thumb is at a natural 45⁰ angle. Now that you have become familiar with the working edge of the thumb, let's *walk* the thumb; it's the secret of using the thumb technique successfully. But before we walk the thumb, let's learn the secret of a successful walk: the bending of the first joint of the thumb. You can demonstrate this to yourself by holding your thumb below the first joint and then bending the top joint. That's the important action you will be using.

Now, taking away your hand from the first joint of your thumb, try to make the thumb bend as before. Place the hand back on the table with the thumb in the natural position and with a steady, even pressure, walk the thumb by slightly bending and unbending the first joint . . . it will "creep" forward in this natural position. We advise against straightening the thumb all the way for it allows too much flat thumb surface to come in contact with the foot thus missing the critical reflexes. (*See Figure 4.3*)

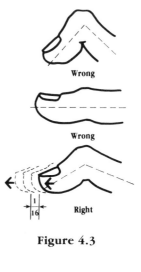

Figure 4.3

37

While this thumb walking is a very important part of the technique in applying successful Reflexology theory, you will be combining it with an equally important and naturally acquired phenomenon called *leverage.* An important fact to remember is that leverage can be obtained by using slight, even pressure with the four fingers of the working hand in opposition to the thumb. The foot is between the thumb and the four fingers.

LEVERAGE

As an example of leverage, place your right thumb on your left forearm and do the walking motion not letting the fingers touch the arm. Now, place the fingers of your working hand firmly underneath the arm for leverage in opposition to your thumb and do the walking motion with your thumb letting the fingers follow along as you move.

Notice how much more pressure you have. This is leverage!

Now that we have discussed the basic thumb technique and the necessary leverage, let's walk the thumb. Remember, we want to walk the thumb by bending the first joint and taking small, tiny bites. It is necessary when learning this technique to practice, practice, practice until you feel an even steady pressure. This is not an intermittent pressure, but a steady pressure as the thumb bends like a snail who leaves an even steady trail.

Let's practice walking the thumb on an area of the foot. It is best to practice the thumb technique by working the center of the foot since it is soft and pliant and doesn't require a lot

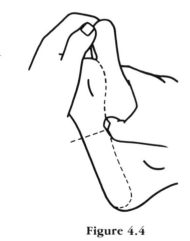

Figure 4.4

of pressure. This also gives you an opportunity to learn the holding hand technique in this area. Remember, the holding hand is going to be used to hold the foot still or *control* it. In this instance, gently grasping the toes and holding them back (***See Figure 4.4***), opens up the area and allows the thumb to easily reach the reflex area. Now you can practice the thumb technique on the bottom of the foot by applying a constant steady pressure, using the corner of the thumb. Another hint for the thumb technique: the thumb always walks forward and never backs up or goes sideways.

While you are practicing walking the thumb in that soft area of the foot, check how much leverage your fingers are providing. You will notice as you work the area you must keep your fingers in the natural holding position or you lose the leverage. The thumb and fingers must be opposite each other to get maximum leverage. Let the leverage fingers follow along as you work; don't let them get too far away so that the hand is stretched out as your hands will become fatigued.

This is the basic thumb technique. Upon this technique, you will be building your whole career as a Reflexologist. And, as in any science, practice is going to pay off and as you begin to develop your Reflexology techniques you will be able to *target in* on the reflex areas so necessary for a successful treatment.

Another thing you may notice as you begin is that while working or practicing, an area of the thumb or that joint on the thumb may become a little sore. Just as in developing any muscle (as any athlete can affirm) it takes time to build strength and it takes a lot of practice. Remember to maintain constant pressure as your thumb walks forward. A good idea would be to test your thumb technique on your arm. The real test is a feeling of constant pressure much as if someone were drawing a line down the arm with a felt tip pen. If this steady pressure is not evident and there is more of a feeling of *on and off* pressure, then review the technique including the bending of that first joint. (**See Figure 4.5**).

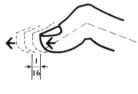

Figure 4.5

As you review this technique, keep in mind that you are working on the basic rule to effectively work the reflex areas. You must maintain that steady constant pressure and the necessary leverage. It is leverage that gives your thumb the strength as you work the reflex areas of the foot. The angle that you use your thumb aids your total leverage as well.

THE FINGER TECHNIQUE

The second technique that a Reflexologist learns is basically the same as the thumb technique in that we will be using an area of the finger in conjunction with the bending of the first joint of that finger. We will be using the inside edge of the finger just as we use the inside edge of the thumb.

This time, in the finger technique, leverage is obtained by use of the thumb when it is opposed to the fingers.

As in all Reflexology operating modes, the finger technique needs constant practice. The object of that practice is the same as with the thumb technique: taking creeping motions by smaller and smaller *bites* and exerting a constant and

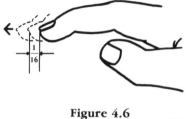

Figure 4.6

steady forward pressure. Once again, we do not want the on-and-off type of pressure. And, as with the thumb, the finger always moves in a forward direction, never back or sideways. (*See* *Figure 4.6*)

It is also important to remember that only one finger does the actual walking. As a rule, we will be using the index finger for most of these techniques. As the fingers are generally narrower, we use them to work certain areas which could not be worked as effectively by using the thumbs, also, it will rest our thumbs during a treatment.

40

Now, of course, one finger cannot walk off by itself without taking the other fingers along, so the other fingers help with the leverage of the index finger. Your first difficulty in executing the finger technique will probably involve bending the first joint of the finger. Practice by holding the index finger just behind its first joint and then bending the first joint only. Other things to avoid as you practice are scratching or digging the fingernail into the skin; sometimes reversing or allowing the fingers to draw back and burn the skin rather than a forward constant pressure; some people merely roll the finger from side to side. These difficulties can be overcome only with practice, practice, practice.

Only the first joint of the finger or thumb is flexed and not too high for three reasons: 1) it will cause too much stress on the joint of person giving treatment; 2) the person receiving treatment will feel your nails; and 3) you will miss a lot of contact with the skin.

When working an area, we must keep the working finger or thumb parallel to the surface being worked on and at a slight angle taking small *bites*. When working many areas of the foot, such as the spine and sinus reflexes, the fingers are used to give the working thumb leverage and smoothness throughout the whole operation.

A tender reflex must be worked from several directions: up, down and across. Very often, walking over an area in one direction will not elicit any sensitivity, but coming back in the opposite direction will many times be quite sensitive. The reason for this direction response is not exactly understood it is possible that the subcutaneous granulations that we sometimes feel and work on are laid down in layers. Try to feel any changes in the tissues on which contact is being made, i.e., granulations, changes of tension or just a difference in feel.

THE THUMB "HOOK-IN, BACK-UP" TECHNIQUE or "BUMBLEBEE ACTION"

As you progress through your Reflexology techniques and begin to understand the anatomy associated with working Reflexology, you will soon discover that there are certain target areas that the Reflexologist must work which call for *pinpoint* accuracy. When it comes to pinpoint accuracy, you will use the *hook-in, back-up* technique. I have termed this the *bumblebee* technique. Any of you who have been subjected to a sting of that little insect are probably aware of its habit of implanting the stinger into your anatomy. He lands on your arm and backs up the stinger into your flesh. This is basically the action your thumb is going to use. You're going to hook it in and back it up.

Just as you did using the thumb technique, you must bend the first joint of the thumb and exert pressure with the inside corner of the thumb. Once you have placed the thumb on a reflex point on the foot, you push in and pull back across

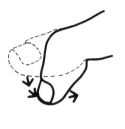

Figure 4.7

the point with the thumb just as that bee lands on a spot and backs that stinger into your flesh, the thumb will emulate the same motion. It will *hook-in and back-up.* (***See Figure 4.7.***) Be sure when you use this technique not to slide across the surface of the skin but keep the thumb in contact and only move the underlying tissue.

Since this technique calls for pinpointing and usually the area represents deep points within the body; leverage is extremely important. For the hook-in and back-up technique, we use the wrist as well as the fingers for leverage.

We use the term pinpointing since there is no *walking* with the thumb. You are landing on a small point hooking in and backing up.

"REFLEX ROTATION" or "PIVOT POINT" TECHNIQUE

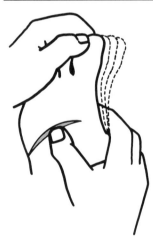

Figure 4.8

Reflex rotation technique is a valuable aid in working particularly tender areas. Once the area is pinpointed, we're going to put pressure on this area with the thumb. With the holding hand, grasp the foot in a comfortable position and flex the foot slowly into the thumb with the holding hand. Flex several times; this gives increased pressure at the reflex point. Then slowly shift the pressure thumb around the region, only working to the discomfort tolerance of the person. Watch out for digging in with your fingernail. This technique can be done with either hand and is ideally adapted for use when working on your own feet. (***See Figure 4.8***).

NOTE: Some of the techniques which I have described can be administered to your own feet and can be very effective, limited, of course, by your own agility.

DISCOMFORT

We must remember that when giving a treatment, the idea is not to cause unnecessary discomfort. The face of the person receiving treatment must always be watched and pressure adjusted as necessary. What we must work for is an indicative sign, almost what a trained Reflexologist calls, *relaxing pain*. Yes, there is such a thing.

RELAXING TECHNIQUES

BACK AND FORTH

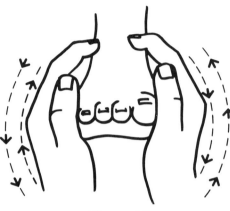

Figure 4.9

Place the palm of your hands, one on the inside and one on the outside edge of the metatarsal padding and then move your hands rapidly back and forth with your fingers relaxed (*the hands will be going in the opposite direction from each other*). Be sure your hands are held firmly against the foot so as not to burn the skin of the foot. (*See Figure 4.9*). But when you relax your fingers and allow them to lightly slap the top of the foot, it will add to the relaxing sensation.

METATARSAL KNEADING

Wrap your right hand around the top of the foot with the index finger just below the base of the toes. Your left hand

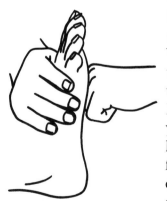

Figure 4.10

will be made into a fist and placed flatly against the bottom of the foot directly opposite the right hand. Work the hands in a kneading motion. Push your fist against the foot, then as you squeeze with the other hand release a little pressure with your fist. When using this technique, keep both hands in contact with the foot at all times. When one hand is either pushing or squeezing, the other hand is just slightly relaxed. You may also alternate the hands for this procedure. (*See Figure 4.10.*)

SPINAL TWIST

Place your hands together with your palms down and index fingers touching each other; your thumbs will also be down. With the foot tipped out, place your two hands as a unit firmly around the foot with the webbing of the thumbs and fingers placed on the spinal reflex area and the thumbs on the bottom of the foot. The center of the two hands will be just below the guideline to the waist. The two hands should be used as a unit keeping all the fingers together and the two hands touching at all times. The hand close to the heel will remain stationary while the other hand will rotate slowly and smoothly back and forth. After several rotations, move the two hands together gradually inching up toward the toes and continue the rotation remembering to keep the hand toward the heel stationary at all times. Continue this process until the hand toward the toes is over the great toe. Be sure when you rotate the foot that you twist the foot evenly in both directions. (*See Figure 4.11*.)

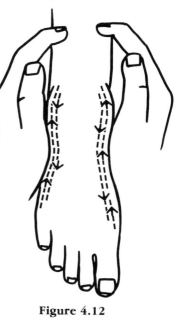

Figure 4.11

ANKLE LOOSENING

Place the heel of your hands below the ankle bone, one on the inside and one on the outside, then move your hands rapidly back and forth (*the hands will be going in the opposite direction from each other*). The foot will shake from side to side. Be sure your hands are kept firmly against the

Figure 4.12

foot so as not to burn the skin. (*See Figure 4.12*.) After you become adept at this maneuver, you can try to slowly roll the

45

heel of your hands from the outside edge to the inside edge and then back as you rapidly move them back and forth.

ANKLE ROTATION "UNDER"

Rest the right heel in the palm of the left hand, hold the middle finger of the left hand gently on the uterus/prostate reflex area. The thumb of the left hand will wrap around the outside part of the ankle where the leg is joined onto the

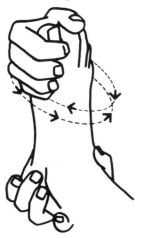

foot (groin reflex). Next, place the heel of the right hand on the bottom of the foot at the metatarsal area with the fingers gently wrapped over the toes and then rotate the foot back and forth in a slight oval motion four or five times in one direction and the same number of times in the other direction while controlling the pressure with the middle finger. Repeat this process on the left foot with the alternate hands. Besides being a relaxation technique, this is also working the reflex to the uterus and the prostate. (*See Figure 4.13*.)

Figure 4.13

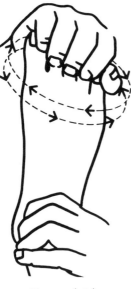

Figure 4.14

ANKLE ROTATION "OVER"

Place the left hand with the fingers together over the top of the foot with the webbing between the thumb and fingers over the ankle joint where the foot is joined onto the leg (groin area). The rest of the fingers are firmly wrapped around the leg. Place the heel of the right hand on the bottom of the foot at the metatarsal area with the fingers gently wrapped over the toes and rotate the foot in a slight oval motion several times in one direction, then several times in the other direction. (*See Figure 4.14*.)

TOE ROTATION

With the thumb and fingers of the left hand, firmly hold the base of the toe you wish to rotate. Take your thumb and first two fingers of your right hand and place them over the toe all the way to its base. With a slight lift, rotate each toe first in one direction several times, then in the opposite direction the same number of times. (*See Figure 4.15*.)

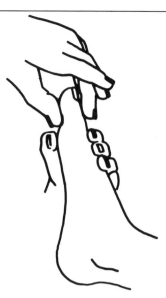

Figure 4.15

DIAPHRAGM—DEEP BREATHING

Place the ball of your thumbs in the center of the diaphragm/solar plexus reflex on both feet at the same time, allowing the fingers to comfortably lay on the top of the foot. Ask your client to take a deep breath and hold it each time you press on this reflex. You should push on this reflex as they take a deep breath and hold the pressure while they hold their breath for a short time. As they slowly exhale, you should slowly let up on the pressure about half-way. Do this four or five times gradually increasing the time you hold the pressure and they hold their breath. Always maintain about half the pressure when they slowly exhale. It helps if you breathe with them. (*See Figure 4.16*.) This technique is generally reserved for the end of a session.

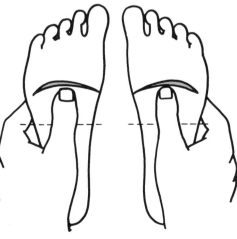

Figure 4.16

DIAPHRAGM—TENSION RELAXER

In this relaxing technique, you will work the whole diaphragm reflex area by starting at the inside edge of the foot below the metatarsals. Place your working thumb on the reflex with a slight angle up under the metatarsals. With

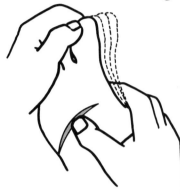

the holding hand, grasp the toes, lift slightly, and pull the foot toward you . . . this will pull the foot onto the thumb. Your thumb should then take one small step toward the outside and repeat the process. Continue until you reach the outside edge. Change hands and work toward the inside edge. This is extremely effective for a tense person or one with hypertension (high blood pressure). (*See Figure 4.17.*)

Figure 4.17

INTRODUCTION TO THE SYSTEMS

The human body is composed of a myriad of parts working together for the good health of the entire being. These parts are usually grouped into systems: structures and organs related to each other in performing certain functions.

In the following chapters, each of these systems including their functions and integral parts are briefly described. This is followed by a detailed discussion concerning the reflex points of the components of these systems, their locations on the feet and the exact techniques used to work these reflexes.

In order to be a good Reflexologist one must understand each system of the body more fully. Do not restrict your study to just this volume. Anatomy and physiology of the human body require continual study as we are always learning new things.

We will be describing these procedures system by system. In our seminars we have found that this is the best method for learning. This, however, would not be the suggested order for giving a Reflexology session. For the proper sequence see Chapter 14.

As most components of a system are found on both feet, we will simplify things by describing how to work on the system's reflex points on the right foot throughout this book. It should be noted that in working these reflexes I will start with the right hand as the working hand as I begin to work on the right foot. When the reflex for a specific organ is located only on the left foot, I will then work the left foot.

All of the reflexes associated with the systems are illustrated on the fold out chart located at the back of this book. The chart may be folded out for visibly studying it while reading the chapters.

Chapter 5

THE SKELETAL, NERVOUS, AND MUSCULAR SYSTEMS

"From whom the whole body fitly joined together and compacted by that which every joint supplieth . . ."

Ephesians 4:16

THE SKELETAL, NERVOUS AND MUSCULAR SYSTEM

As you practice Reflexology more and more, you will see that these three systems are so intimately related and interconnected that it would be beyond the scope of this book to divide and delve into each of the three. That task remains the challenge of the writers of anatomy books as well as those of the neurophysiologists.

However, I will touch upon some basic anatomy, nerve and muscle functions and suggest that you become familiar with some of the more prominent muscles as well as nerve plexus and bones. I would particularly recommend your becoming familiar with the bones of the foot since some of them are used for reference points throughout this book.

As a handy guide and suitable reference book which gives an excellent overview and introduction to the systems, I always recommend to my students **The Atlas of Human Anatomy**, published by Barnes and Noble Books. Another one which is quite detailed and which you might find interesting is **Structure and Function in Man**, published by W. B. Saunders Company. Both are useful adjuncts to the serious student of Reflexology.

One thing I might add here is the thought that, as you study these three systems or, as a matter of fact, as you study all the systems of the body, it should become abundantly clear that the human body is truly a work of divine creation.

THE SKELETAL SYSTEM

Here is an assemblage of one of the busiest tissues in the body, a veritable chemical factory that is constantly busy and involved in processes which include the production of blood components, minerals and other vital materials. We don't usually think of our skeletal system in that way. Most of us think of the bones as supporting the body and affording protection for the organs. . . 206 bones with the *neck bone connected to the shoulder bones*, and so on as the old song goes. Well, it is true that the skeletal system **does** support and protect, but it also contributes a whole lot more to our well being. (**See Figure 5.1**)

As a matter of fact, we seldom think of the bones as organs, but they are when you consider the medical definition of an organ as *"a somewhat independent part of the body that performs a special function or functions."*

Look at it this way: Bones act as a reservoir for most of the body's mineral needs including:

99% of the calcium

88% of the phosphorus, plus copper and cobalt.

And these structural *factories* work around the clock making the cellular elements of the blood.

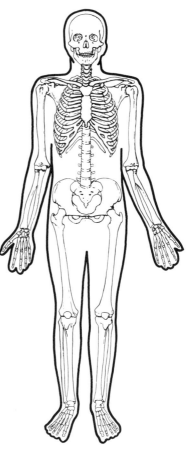

Figure 5.1

When you consider that this body of yours uses up or depletes 180-million red blood cells in a single minute, and that the bones resupply most of their replacements, then you begin to see just how important those 206 bones are. In the bone marrow, red, white and platelet cells are manufactured every day. And the bones also contain millions of cells called osteoblasts which produce a highly important form of protein called collagen, the matrix for new bone that is constantly being replenished in the body.

Then consider that all important mineral: calcium. It is released into the body from the bones when needed to supply vital functions. This is a very critical role which keeps a delicate balance in the body's chemical factory.

Last but not least, the bones serve as moorings for muscles. We would move nowhere if our muscles were not attached to bones via tendons and ligaments . . . those tough bands of connective tissue which hold those 206 bones and muscles together.

These connecting parts, the tendons and ligaments, are prone to injury, especially when they are used inappropriately and when one's nutrition is subpar. Thus, we experience strains and sprains. The Reflexologist must always consider the role that these tendons and ligaments play in injuries to the skeletal system.

I should also mention *articulations*. The word is used to describe the connection of bone to bone within the skeletal system and is usually divided into *movable* and *immovable* joints. The thing to remember here is that the movable joints contain a cavity filled with a joint lubricating fluid called *synovia*. The cavity containing the fluid is called a *bursa*. When the bursa of a joint of the great toe becomes inflamed, it thickens, the joint enlarges and sometimes *displaces* or makes the toe crooked . . . then we have a *bunion*.

While on the subject of bones, it is important that the Reflexologist note the striking similarity and relationship of the shoulder to the hip, and the arm to the leg. We will be discussing these *referral areas* later when we talk about *working the reflexes* in this chapter.

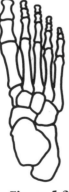

Figure 5.2

THE FOOT

Almost one-fourth of all bones in the entire human body are located in the feet (*See Figure 5.2*). Each foot is composed of twenty-six (26) bones assembled into what has been called one of the most fantastic engineering accomplishments of all time. Twenty-six bones, 107 ligaments and 19 muscles of each foot support and balance the rest of the body.

If we think of our feet as the foundation of our home, then we get a pretty good picture of just how important they are. If we don't have a solid foundation, the whole structure suffers. We know that when the feet are out of alignment, it can create a situation conducive to many health problems. For instance, if you walk favoring one foot over the other, you almost invariably throw the back out of alignment. Conversely, if the back or spine is out of alignment, you sometimes will walk favoring one side of the body and one foot, which leads to foot problems.

THE BONES OF THE FOOT

Some of the bones of the foot are of particular interest to the Reflexologist, including the tarsal bones which compare to the wrist bones. These are seven in number and are in the heel and back part of the foot. The five long bones (the metatarsals), and the 14 bones (phalanges) of the toes correspond to the metacarpals of the hand and the phalanges of the fingers and thumbs, respectively. Get to know these bones of the foot, you will find that *familiarity breeds contentment*.

57

THE NERVOUS SYSTEM

No system in the human body exemplifies homeostasis better than the nervous system . . . every cell of every nerve fiber must work in balance for maximum performance. The nervous system is the intricate *link* to all systems of the human body. It can be compared to the wiring system of your house . . . when all the appliances work and the air conditioner or the heater is making life comfortable, we give little thought to that mass of wires, fuses and switches that are responsible for our feeling of well-being. But let something happen to that system and then we realize just how important those things are. The main components of this system are, of course, the brain and the spinal cord.

THE BRAIN (*see figure 5.3*)

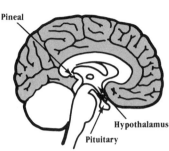

Pineal

Hypothalamus

Pituitary

Figure 5.3

It has been estimated that an electron tube computer would have to be the size of a New York City skyscraper to contain the equipment comparable to that in the three pounds or so of the human brain.

Every cell in the body is ruled by the brain . . . dreaming, speaking, thinking . . . even *changing our mind*.

Nearly 2500 years ago, Hippocrates, after studying head wounds, concluded that *the brain of man is double*, an astute observation, since the brain is composed of two symmetrical hemispheres. The left hemisphere of the brain controls the right side of the body while the right hemisphere controls the left side. This is the reason why, when someone is paralyzed on the right side, it is the left portion of the brain that has been damaged.

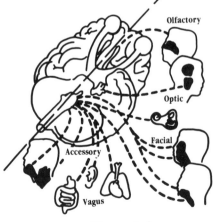

Olfactory

Optic

Facial

Accessory

Vagus

Figure 5.4

The medulla is called the *control center* of the brain as well as the *switchboard* since it is from this area that the twelve (12) pairs of cranial nerves arise. These cranial nerves *connect* the body to the brain serving the sensory and motor needs of head, neck, chest, and abdomen. (*See Figure 5.4*).

Basically, the brain functions in many different ways:

- **It regulates** body activities as well as controlling them. It adjusts the body's mechanism for changes to internal or external conditions.

- It is the **center of consciousness**. It makes you aware of time and place, etc.

- It is the **seat of sensations**. It receives impulses from the sense organs: eyes, ears, nose, etc., and turns them into sensations of sight, hearing, smell, touch, etc.

- It is the **source of voluntary acts**.

- It is the **seat of our emotions**.

- It is the **center for thought**, **reasoning**, **memory** . . . all the so-called higher mental processes.

- And, it sits on another important **life line** . . . the spine.

THE SPINE — LIFE LINE OF THE BODY

The spine is the center of the body and the center of more trouble and misery than almost any other structure you carry around in your being. That's probably because that articulated hollow group of odd-shaped bones is put under stress when you stand erect (and have all that weight bearing down upon it). And look what you make it do . . . bend, swivel, twist and contort to a point where it almost screams *enough*. Only when it has had more than enough does it let you know by the so-called *slipped disc*, lower back pain, etc.

Yet, this engineering marvel we call the spine has to be taken seriously if we realize that the hollow center carries a nerve system that would put any telephone company to shame. The spinal cord carries millions of messages back and forth from the brain and body . . . every conceivable motion you make is the result of an instantaneous message flashed through that direct line . . . 31 pairs of nerves transmitting constantly. The spinal cord is protected against shock with a unique *shock absorber* called cerebrospinal fluid (CSF) and, of course, the bones or vertebrae which protect the whole system. But it doesn't even stop there ... these vertebrae are able to twist and bend because

59

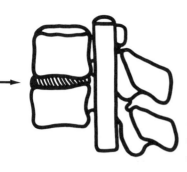

they are *padded*. Each of these oddly-shaped bones rest on *pads* or *discs* (**See Figure 5.5**) which are covered with a tough membranous envelope.

Figure 5.5

Acting as another natural *shock absorber* of the spine are the strange *curves* themselves. The spinal curves are designed in such a way that they actually absorb the daily shock that results from walking, running, or jogging . . . or even lifting that bag of groceries from the back of the car. Hundreds of muscles and almost a thousand ligaments are a constant working part of this system. Stress and tension can affect all of them or a series of them, enough to make *backache* a common household word.

Before we begin looking into the physiology and anatomy of the spine, it is interesting to note just how the spine relates to the structure of the feet.

The adult spine consists of 26 vertebrae; the feet have 26 bones. The adult spine has four curves: the sacral, lumbar, thoracic and the cervical. Each foot has four curves.

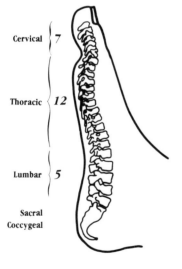

Cervical 7

Thoracic 12

Lumbar 5

Sacral
Coccygeal

Figure 5.6

When I speak of the curves of the foot, I am referring to those curves along the medial longitudinal arch. If we place these curves against a lateral view of the spine, we can easily see how the curves of the spine match the curves of the feet (**See Figure 5.6**).

The spine, or vertebral column, is a part of the axial skeleton. It is a strong, flexible, rod-like structure which supports the head, gives attachments to the ribs, and encloses and protects the vital spinal cord.

The vertebrae are divided into five groups according to their distinguishing characteristics. The cervical region has seven vertebrae; the thoracic region, twelve; the lumbar, five; the sacral, one; and the coccyx is made up of fused vertebrae. These vertebrae are all separated by discs which are cushion-like structures that serve to absorb shock. They have a tough envelope of cartilage containing a jelly-like substance.

We hear so much these days about low back pain. It is an international plague. Many back pain sufferers attribute low back pain to a slipped disc. Most of the time, however, low back pain has other origins such as weak muscles, asymmetrical posture, overweight, osteoporosis, and many other conditions. Many conditions in the low back including some forms of sciatica are helped in the alleviation of discomfort by Reflexology.

The spine is supported by hundreds of muscles and ligaments. Lack of proper exercise, stress of life, and poor posture are responsible for most of today's back problems.

Without exercise, these muscles will weaken, and sitting over an office desk or slumping in an arm chair watching television will produce uneven stress throughout the entire length of the spine.

"Structure Governs Function" is a common saying among osteopathic physicians. This is easy to understand when we realize that there are 31 pairs of spinal nerves from the base of the brain. They come out from the spinal cord and connect to the various organs, glands and structures throughout the entire body. The body's vital functions depend on an unimpeded nerve supply as well as adequate blood supply if it is to perform at optimum level. When we study this awesome, complex network, we can readily understand the vital importance of *"Structures Governing Function."*

ABNORMAL TENSION OF MUSCLE OR LIGAMENTS upon any vertebra or group of vertebrae will cause pressure upon a spinal nerve which supplies, for instance, the liver or kidneys. This pressure even though slight, may be enough over a period of time, sometimes even many years, to reduce nerve supply and circulation to those organs.

This spinal tension is caused by stress, **mental or physical**, but acts like a tourniquet upon the affected part whose function will be affected to a lesser or greater degree, but, in any instance, enough to affect homeostasis.

We can say here that since most back pain is associated with tension, we have in Reflexology a very valuable modality in that one of its prime benefits is the reduction of tension or stress. Another point to remember is that we do not just work the spinal reflex areas for conditions associated with back pain . . . we should work these reflex areas often during any Reflexology session. This way, we are able to reduce any tension along the spine which would optimize the nerve and blood supply to other important parts of the body.

We must always keep in mind that the spine is regarded as **one** organ. With that in mind, it is easy to see that whatever affects one end of it will also have an affect on the other end, and vice-versa. We must always work the entire spinal reflex.

Also, don't forget to include the spine helper areas which are the hip/sciatic; hip/knee/leg; side of neck, and the shoulder.

THE MUSCULAR SYSTEM

Many times I am asked why my discussion of the muscular system is included with that of the skeletal system. The reason is obvious since the two systems are so closely tied together in enabling the body to have locomotion and body posture as well as manipulation of the fingers, the eyes, the tongue, etc.

For our purposes here, we will define the muscular system as that part of the body that contracts and relaxes giving the body movement and posture. Besides the muscles themselves, we are going to include the tendons and ligaments.

Muscle functions are usually divided into two kinds: voluntary and involuntary.

While sometimes this division of muscle function is hazy, let's accept the definition and look at the functions this way.

The voluntary functions include the maintenance of proper posture and those movements which are readily visible, including the limbs and fingers. The toes play an important part in balance and locomotion. The diaphragm which is a large umbrella-shaped muscular band is necessary for respiration; as the pharynx is needed for swallowing. The tongue and lips enable us to eat and speak; the abdominal wall assists in breathing and elimination. All of these muscular structures are under voluntary control.

Involuntary muscular functions include the movement of food through the digestive tract called peristalsis. It also includes the movement of bile from the gall bladder, urine from the kidneys, and the contractions of the uterus. Other involuntary functions include the regulation of the size of openings in the pupil of the eye or the neck of the bladder. And then there is the opening of blood vessels and the bronchioles in the lungs . . . all of them regulated without our even trying.

A few words about *fatigue*.

All of us have experienced this tired sensation which is often felt in the muscles. It is usually defined as the inability of the muscle to perform work. There are several factors which are responsible for this type of sensation . . . some:

- Excessive activity: this is a definite cause of fatigue and rest will cure it.

- Inadequate activity: this often goes unrecognized; it underlies the fact that most persons feel better when they exercise.

- Malnutrition: caused by a lack of proper foods, especially needed are proteins, minerals and vitamins.

- Circulatory disturbances: when not enough oxygen, glucose and nutrients get to the muscles and when the blood cannot remove waste products, fatigue occurs in the affected muscles.

- Respiratory disturbance: when the oxygen/carbon dioxide ratio is upset as in emphysema.

- Infections: cause fatigue since the energies of the body are used to fight the infection.

- Endocrine gland disturbances: as seen in menopause, diabetes, thyroid, and adrenal disorders.

- Other factors include poor posture and some cases of eyestrain.

THE EFFECT OF EXERCISE ON THE MUSCULAR SYSTEM

Activity as found in a sound program of exercise brings about a profound effect on the muscles of the body; but even more importantly, nearly every other system of the body is affected too. Heart rate, respiration, perspiration, and the skeletal framework all respond to exercise. The ability of the muscles to take up and utilize oxygen depends upon their use. As I always say, *"what we don't use . . . we lose."* So a planned program of regular exercise is a must for full performance of bodily systems.

WORKING THE SKELETAL, NERVOUS, AND MUSCULAR SYSTEMS

In selecting a working sequence for this section, it was only natural that I should follow the subject of our discussion. . . the anatomy of the body. So, we will begin with the highest structure, of course, the brain and then work through the spine and the muscles to the feet.

WORKING THE BRAIN

The main focal areas for working the brain are the tips of the great toes, since each represents one-half of the head. This, of course, does not exclude the tips of the small toes since they aid in *fine-tuning* anything in the head.

We will hold the right great toe with the left hand. The index finger of the right hand will be used to work across the tip of the great toe in a rolling motion. (*See Figure 5.7*). You will start with the outside edge of the tip of your index finger on the outside edge of the tip (just below the toenail) of the great toe. You will roll the finger with the pressure downward from the outside edge of the inside; pick it up and move to where you finished and repeat this process until the entire tip of the great toe is covered. Repeat this entire process several times on the right foot and then still using the right hand, work the left great toe in the same manner.

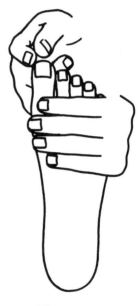

65

Figure 5.7

WORKING THE SPINE

The following guidelines are of great importance in order for us to accurately locate certain vertebrae. This is quite understandable since we are all unique in our physical make-up.

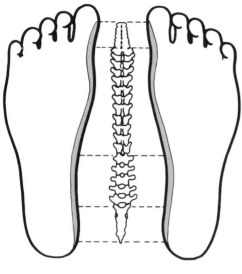

The reflex areas for the spine are located on the inside edge of both feet ... the right foot corresponding to the right side of the spine; the left foot to the left side of the spine. (***See Figure 5.8***).

When working the spinal reflex areas, I recommend working up and down them each time, thus covering a slightly different portion of the spine; the reason becomes evident when we realize the spine is a relatively wide structure. Also,

Figure 5.8

you must be sure that you work **across** each of these areas. The heel of the holding hand will be on the metatarsals of the foot with the fingers wrapped around the toes when working **up** the spine. When working **down** the spine, the heel of the foot is resting in the opposite hand.

66

SACRUM—COCCYX REFLEX

One of the most difficult reflexes to work is the sacrum-coccyx reflex located in the heel area . . . normally a callused area of thick, tough skin which simply indicates that more pressure than usual is needed to adequately work this region.

It is here, at the sacrum and coccyx, on the lower end of the spine where many injuries are manifested. The lower lumbar is important, too. It is an *inherent weakness* in many people and *lower back pain* is a constant source of distress. As a matter of fact, there are very few of us who haven't injured our back at one time or another. And when we do injure a certain area, there is a build-up that occurs from the trauma so you will usually find that the lower back reflex area will be sensitive on most people. While this does not necessarily indicate serious problems in all cases, it may reflect congestion possibly from previous injuries. As I so often have stated in my seminars: remember, if one end of the spine is affected, it often affects the opposite end. As we work the lower portion of the spine, it will often help the neck region and many headaches that are caused by lower back problems.

The spine remains a vital area to the Reflexologist, and especially the lower back for such conditions as migraine headache, constipation, prostate and female disorders. Many times these are manifestations of stress or tension which have "settled" in the spine.

After all, the spine is the center of the body's equilibrium as it holds us erect. And that spine is surrounded by muscles, ligaments, tendons and a great many nerves. When tension builds up and perhaps pulls a set of muscles, we have the entire body reacting to fight that tension. Some people describe it as *"their back being out"*. . . it is simply muscles pulling on that spine as a result of tension. Certainly, subluxations may occur meaning the vertebrae are out of proper alignment. But remember, bones don't move by themselves—only when pulled by muscles, muscles that are tense, more tense than they should be.

67

The coccyx-sacral reflex area is located in a section of the foot from the back of the heel to the heel guideline on the inside edge of each foot. When working this portion of the foot, as previously mentioned, you will usually find that the skin is tough and callused; this is one of those special areas where **leverage** is so important. Using the fingers of the working hand around the outside of the heel for leverage gives the hand firmness and authority as well as facilitating a smooth, even pressure on this reflex.

At the coccyx-sacral area, I start on the right foot with the heel of the left holding hand against the metatarsals and the fingers lightly over the toes. I use the right thumb and begin to *walk* up the spine reflex from the base of the heel.

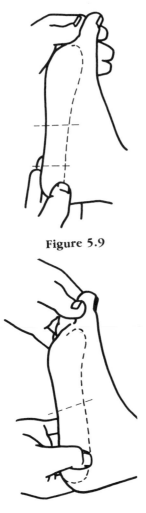

Figure 5.9

Figure 5.10

(**See Figure 5.9**). Note how the fingers of my working hand are placed under the heel of the foot in order to obtain the needed leverage. Next, I work across this spinal reflex area. (**See Figure 5.10**). Then, using my left thumb, I work this same reflex area down to the bottom of the heel as shown in **Figure 5.11**.

Another useful method for extra contact is to use the third finger instead of the thumb to walk up from the base of the heel. (**See Figure 5.12**). We can only walk up a short way with this method, but it is very effective in giving a lot of extra strength to this tough area. When working the sacrum-coccyx area, we must realize we are working the base of the spine. Apart from working for low back pain, we also contact the nerve supply to the pelvic area for conditions such as constipation, bladder problems, prostate disorders, and female problems; in fact, any structure that has nerve innervation from this part of the spine may be affected.

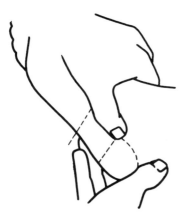

Figure 5.11

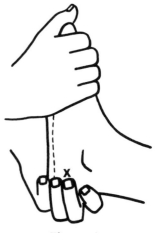

Figure 5.12

LUMBAR REFLEX

Once we have located the heel guideline (*found where the different color of the skin of the heel begins*) we find the location of the fifth lumbar (**See Figure 5.13**). From this point up to the next guideline, the waist, is the lumbar area which is of great importance in working for back pain and for consequent benefit to all the structures in the abdominal area.

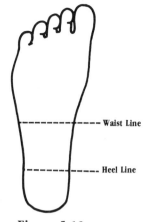

Waist Line

Heel Line

Figure 5.13

Most injuries to the lower spine will involve the fourth to fifth lumbar vertebrae because these support more of the body weight than any of the others.

Also sciatic pain is helped by working the lumbars and sacral reflexes thoroughly, as the sciatic nerve originates from the fourth to fifth lumbar and the sacral, and is the largest nerve in the body.

When I walk up the spine reflex with the thumb, I must change my grip and place the fingers of my working hand over the instep (**See Figure 5.14**). This will then enable me to continue working up to the top of the spine without putting undue stress on my thumb joint.

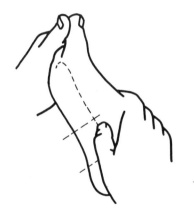

Figure 5.14

69

Then I change hands and work down from the waistline to the heel, as well as working across the reflex. I then reverse this procedure when working the opposite foot with the alternate hand. The helper areas for these regions are very important and include the hip/sciatic reflex and the hip/knee reflex (**See Figure 5.15**).

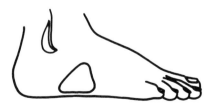

Figure 5.15

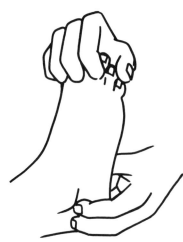

Figure 5.16

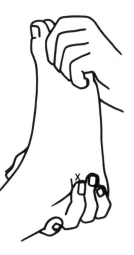

Figure 5.17

HIP/SCIATIC REFLEX

To work this reflex, I will hold the right foot with my right hand. The heel of my right hand will be placed on the metatarsal with my fingers wrapped gently over the toes. (*See* *Figure 5.16*). The fingers are relaxed so as not to squeeze, but still maintaining a slight pressure backward, and with the foot held straight.

I will take my left hand with the palm up and place it under the heel of the right foot with the index finger resting underneath the outside ankle bone and then walk the index finger in a forward motion angling at approximately 45° angle into the ankle bone. I will go approximately ¼ of an inch, stop, lift up, come back and start over. I repeat this process several times. Then I will place the right heel into my right hand; my third finger will be resting in the ankle joint on the outside and I will walk it toward me. (*See Figure 5.17*). This time the left holding hand will be placed on the outside edge of the foot holding the foot straight.

Work approximately ¼ of an inch, stop, lift up, come back and start over, making several passes. Again, the angle is about 45 degrees and you'll be using the inside edge or corner of your finger as it walks underneath that outside ankle bone.

I then repeat this procedure working the opposite foot with the alternate hand. It must be noted that this is a *touchy* reflex and is very sensitive. You **must** keep the foot straight to work it adequately. If you tip the foot toward the inside to see what you are doing (as most people will be tempted to do) this position will tighten up the tendons and will not allow you to reach the reflex area which is sensitive on most people.

This is a helper area for the lower back plus it encompasses the hip and sciatic reflexes. The sciatic nerve is the main nerve which comes through the hip area and down the leg. Remember also that this is a referral area for shoulder problems.

HIP/KNEE/LEG REFLEX

The other helper area for the lower back is the hip/knee/leg reflex area which is located from the fifth metatarsal on the little toe side to the heel on the top of the foot. (**See Figure 5.18**). To work this reflex, our fingers can be used very effectively and thus save our thumb from over-use. Remember: the right holding hand is on the metatarsals and the fingers over the toes. The fingers of my left hand will walk from the outside edge in a forward motion by placing them on the edge around the top part of the foot. I can use my index finger or my middle finger, or simultaneously **use both** fingers to work this area. I could also use my thumb of the same hand (*left hand on the right foot*) on the outside to come up the outer edge in a criss-cross motion. I can also use my alternate hand and come over the top of the foot working toward the outer edge with either thumb or finger. (**See Figure 5.19**). This reflex is found on both feet, an excellent area for hip, knee, and leg problems. This area is *tender* and will usually be extremely sensitive on persons with these problems.

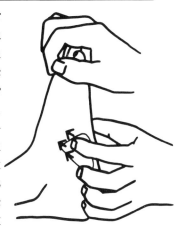

Figure 5.18

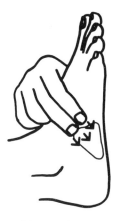

Figure 5.19

Keep these helper areas in mind since they are extremely useful when the lower back is involved.

THORACIC REFLEX

From the waist guideline up to the point where the great toe joins the foot, we have the thoracic part of the spine which is made up of twelve vertebrae. Mental stress can affect this area greatly as well as poor posture. As in any other section or part of the spine, tension can impede nerve supply. Just think of a few of the organs involved in this area: the lungs, heart, liver, spleen, and the kidneys.

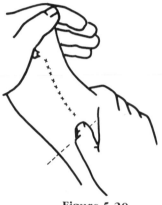

Figure 5.20

The heart, for instance, is supplied by many nerves that originate in the thoracic section of the spine. We can see how important it is to work the spine thoroughly in **every session** to help promote an unimpeded nerve function and not just in the treatment of low back pain. I work both feet the same as for the lumbars: working up, down and across, with my holding hand on the toes. (***See Figure 5.20***).

CERVICAL REFLEX

The seventh cervical is the vertebra that protrudes at the back of the neck and can be easily felt. From the base of the great toe up to the top inside edge opposite the root of the toenail of the great toe is the cervical reflex region. There are seven cervical vertebrae, the top one supports the skull and is called the Atlas and is the first cervical vertebra; the second cervical vertebra is the Axis. All of the facial nerves come off just above the cervicals. The major ones will be the optic, olfactory, vagus, auditory and facial nerves. The lowest cervical vertebra is the seventh cervical. (***See Figure 5.21***). Working the cervicals is always important in the adjunctive treatment of such conditions as ear, eye, nose and facial problems such as Bell's Palsy and Epilepsy.

The sixth and seventh cervical vertebra are important to work in all arm, hand, neck and shoulder problems, including whiplash injury. When working the cervical area, it is best to use the index finger for extra fine treatment.

For the seventh cervical on the right foot, I start at the base of the great toe. I will place my left thumb horizontally across the bottom of the foot on the toes with the fingers on the top of the toes for support. My right index finger will walk around the inside edge of the great toe several times. (*See Figure 5.22*). I can also take my finger and walk toward the tip of the great toe on the inside edge in line with the root of the nail. (*See Figure 5.23*). Next, I take my thumb at the start of the seventh cervical and walk up in the direction of the nail. (*See Figure 5.24*). I shall now use my opposite hand (*left hand, right foot*) at the edge opposite the root of the nail and work down to the base of the great toe. (*See Figure 5.25*). This procedure will be repeated on the left foot.

NOTE: When working the spinal area, we work up and down the reflex area each time covering a slightly different area as the spine is a wide structure. Be sure to work across from the inside to the outside edge of the foot making sure to cross the spinal reflex.

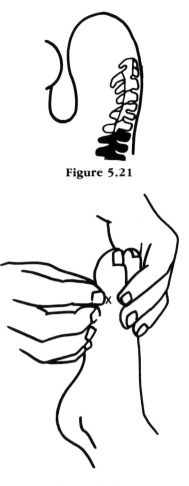

Figure 5.21

Figure 5.22

73

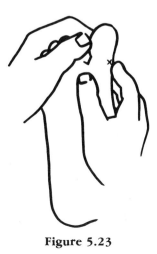

Figure 5.23

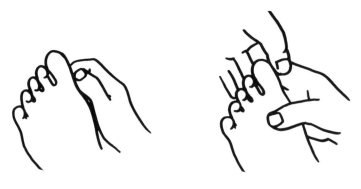

| Figure 5.24 | Figure 5.25 |

When we are working the spine, we will find that *tipping* the foot out is very important. We use our right hand on the right foot and work up the spine reflex. The holding hand will be on the metatarsals with the fingers over the toes. When we work down the spine, we will place our holding hand underneath the heel, and using the left thumb, we work downward using our fingers for leverage. This is true in working all but the cervicals. When working the left foot you will use the opposite hand.

Some common ailments you should be familiar with:

BURSITIS—Inflamation of the bursa. Examples: Tennis Elbow, Housemaid's Knee, bursitis of the shoulder.

When these conditions prevail, spend a little extra time on the reflex to the afflicted area. A helper area would be the adrenal glands.

ARTHRITIS—Enlargement of the bones around the joints.

There are so many causes for arthritis that I will not attempt to limit the areas to be worked. All the reflexes are involved. As with bursitis, a little extra attention should be given to the reflexes to the afflicted areas.

WHIPLASH

An important area, especially for whiplash, is the area between the first and second toe on the top of the foot. It is the best area for whiplash. I start with my right hand on the right foot, my left hand will spread the first and second toes opening up the area. My thumb is in the center of the metatarsal, halfway from the guideline to the diaphragm to the base of the toes—pushing firmly on the metatarsal joint. My index finger of the right hand will walk down at a slight angle in this groove. Keep fingers together for leverage. (*See Figure 5.26*). Walk down several times, making several passes between the great toe and the second toe. Lift, do not drag the finger back. If you bend your finger excessively, you will dig in with the fingernails. Now, repeat this procedure with the left hand. The same technique is used on the left foot.

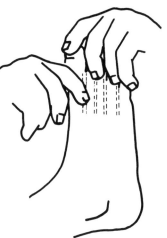

Figure 5.26

SHOULDER REFLEX

Many times neck conditions will affect the shoulder. And the shoulder may affect the neck. Example: If I were to fall on my shoulder, there is a possibility of causing trauma to the neck.

When I work the right shoulder reflex, I'm going to use my left thumb around the little toe joint.

I will keep the foot straight; my right holding hand will be placed on the bottom of the foot, fingers over the toes. My right thumb will be pushing the small toe back and slightly spreading the little toe. This is important as it opens the fourth and fifth metatarsals. My left thumb will start at about the diaphragm line, come around the little toe joint, walking in a forward motion . . . working from the diaphragm line toward the base of the toes. My fingers are wrapped around the top of the foot to give me leverage. I use the side

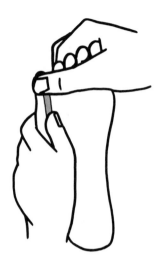

Figure 5.27

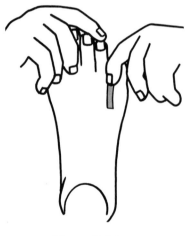

Figure 5.28

of the thumb with basic technique. (**See Figure 5.27**). If you don't push the toes back, the little toe will come forward and not allow you to get into the joint between the 4th and 5th toes. The holding hand is very important to keep on the bottom and to keep the toe pushed back and slightly open, making it easier to work. Never put your holding hand around the top of the foot since this will squeeze the toes. The holding hand is on the bottom, with the heel of the hand on the metatarsals and fingers lightly over the toes.

The shoulder reflex is also a referral area for the hip. I can also work the top of the foot with my index finger on the opposite side from where the thumb worked. (**See Figure 5.28**). My finger will be placed on the top of the foot between the fourth and fifth toes and my thumb will push on the bottom of the foot toward my walking finger. My finger will walk down, starting from the base of the fourth and fifth toes, stop, lift up and work down again. Keep fingers together resting them on the foot for support and leverage. You must maintain pressure on the bottom of the foot, otherwise the foot will *cave in* and you won't have enough finger pressure. Also, I work the outer edge of the little toe joint with the thumb. This area is also for the arm. Repeat process on the left foot with the alternate hand.

AREAS OF THE SPINE AND
THEIR RELATED NERVE INTERVENTIONS

There are thirty-one (31) pairs of nerves which pass through the vertebrae of the spine. These spinal nerves receive sensations from the sense organs and they carry motor instructions to the muscles and glands of the body. Becoming familiar with the spinal nerves, their distribution, and related clinical conditions can be of great help to the Reflexologist. (**See Figure 5.29**).

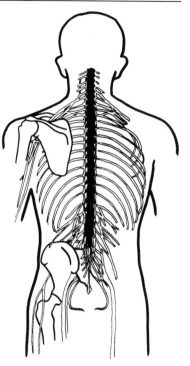

Figure 5.29

CERVICAL AREA

Eight pairs of nerves move through this area and are very influential in affecting areas of the face and head. (There are two coming from the first cervical.)

NERVE	INNERVATION	RELATED CONDITIONS
1st Cervical (2 nerves)	head, pituitary gland, scalp, brain, face, ear	head colds, headaches, amnesia, chronic tiredness, dizziness, muscle tension
2nd Cervical	eyes, sinuses, tongue, forehead, mastoids	sinus trouble, allergies, eye trouble, ear trouble, fainting
3rd Cervical	cheeks, teeth, ears	neuritis, eczema, acne
4th Cervical	nose, lips, mouth, eustachian tube	hay fever, catarrh, blocked eustachian tubes
5th Cervical	neck glands, pharynx, heart	hoarseness, sore throat, etc.

NERVE	INNERVATION	RELATED CONDITIONS
6th Cervical	neck and shoulder muscles, tonsils, heart	stiff neck, pain in the arm, croup, tonsillitis
7th Cervical	thyroid, shoulders and elbows, heart	bursitis, thyroid problems, colds

THE THORACIC AREA

Twelve pairs of nerves pass through this area of the spine and all influence a great number of organs and glands in the upper trunk area; they also have an effect on hands and arms.

NERVE	INNERVATION	RELATED CONDITIONS
1st Thoracic	lower arms from the elbow, wrists, hands and fingers, the esophagus and wind pipe, heart	asthma, coughs, breathing difficulties, pain below the elbows and in the hand
2nd Thoracic	heart and coronary arteries	chest pain and functional heart conditions
3rd Thoracic	lungs, bronchial tubes (respiration area), pleura, chest, heart	pleurisy, pneumonia, the grippe, bronchitis
4th Thoracic	gall bladder and common bile duct, heart	jaundice and gall bladder problems
5th Thoracic	solar plexus, liver, heart	fever, low blood pressure, anemia, arthritis, and adverse liver conditions
6th Thoracic	the stomach	indigestion, heart burn and nervous stomach
7th Thoracic	pancreas, duodenum	ulcers, diabetes and often gastritis

NERVE	INNERVATION	RELATED CONDITIONS
8th Thoracic	spleen and diaphragm	leukemia, hiccoughs
9th Thoracic	adrenal glands	allergies, hives, and an inadequate reaction to stress
10th Thoracic	kidneys	kidney trouble, fatigue, hardening of the arteries
11th Thoracic	kidneys and ureters	skin disorders and autointoxication (absorption of poison from the gastrointestinal canal)
12th Thoracic	small intestines, fallopian tubes and lymph circulation	gas pains, rheumatism, lymphatic congestion

THE LUMBAR, SACRAL AND COCCYX AREAS

This area of the spine has nerves supplying the lower area of the body and the legs.

NERVE	INNERVATION	RELATED CONDITIONS
1st Lumbar	colon and groin area	inflammation of the colon, constipation, hernia and diarrhea
2nd Lumbar	abdomen and its contents, appendix, blind pouch (cecum) and the thighs	cramps, appendicitis, varicose veins, breathing difficulties
3rd Lumbar	reproductive glands, urinary bladder and knee	bladder trouble, painful or irregular menstrual periods, change of life symptoms, knee pains, involuntary discharge of urine, impotency

NERVE	INNERVATION	RELATED CONDITIONS
4th Lumbar	muscles of the lower back, sciatic nerve and the prostate gland	lumbago, backaches, too frequent urination and sciatica. Note: The sciatic is the largest nerve in the body and affects nearly the whole of the leg, muscles of the back of the thigh, and the foot
5th Lumbar	lower legs, ankles, feet, toes and arches	cold feet, weakness and poor circulation in the legs, weak or swollen ankles and leg cramps
The Sacrum	hip bone and buttocks	curvature of the spine and sacroiliac strain
The Coccyx	rectum and anus	hemorrhoids, pain at the end of spine, anal itch

NOTE: In reviewing the spinal chart, it is well to note that very few of the conditions listed here are wholly under the control of any one nerve.

80

IN SUMMARY

The entire body below the neck, including the arms and the legs, is controlled by the spinal cord. Sensations from body parts traverse the spinal nerves, enter the spinal cord, and then are relayed to the brain and other spinal centers. Messages from the cord or from the brain exit via spinal nerves to control the action of blood vessels, muscles and glands. From a simple reflex arc to the most deliberate planned activity, the spinal cord and its nerves serve the body every minute of every day.

Whenever there is impingement or entrapment of spinal nerves, serious body disfunctions may occur. Pressure on nerves may be due to injuries, tight (hypertonic) muscles, fibrotic scar tissue, vertebral subluxations, and other causes.

Reflexology can nudge the body toward better functioning by improving lymphatic drainage, circulation and muscle relaxation. The wise Reflexologist will never forget the spine and its integral effects upon the whole body.

A WORD ON MUSCULAR TENSION

Tension is manifested many times in the trapezius and deltoid muscles of the back and shoulders. A particularly effective Reflexology technique for this specific area has been developed by me through years of practice and work on this widespead affliction.

For tension in the neck muscles, I work the outside of the great toe. For all of the affected areas, including the trapezius and deltoids, I work across the top of the foot from the great toe to the little toe in the metatarsal area, particularly the grooves between the toes.

I generally find it more effective to work the top of the foot although you **can** work the bottom, but, since it is made up of a lot tougher layer of skin, the top seems more effective. However, I would recommend working both **the top and the bottom.**

Tension is also relieved by working the diaphragm reflex area. I work across this area with the standard thumb technique. Another technique we have developed for this area is to put the thumb on this area, then pull the foot **onto** the thumb, move the thumb a bit, stop, pull the foot onto the thumb, etc. Work in this manner across the entire reflex area. (**See Figure 5.30**).

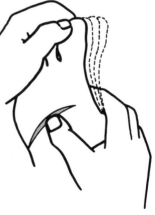

Figure 5.30

For numbness in the arms, hands or feet, I find that working the shoulder reflex often helps.

For lower back and leg complaints, we always work the sciatic nerve reflex. A referral area for leg muscles would be to work the corresponding area on the arm.

A NOTE TO REMEMBER: Whenever you work the muscles, always remember that it is the adrenals that give the body muscles their *tone* . . . always be sure to work the adrenals.

CORNS AND CALLUSES

If a person's spine or hip is out of alignment, this situation can cause corns and calluses. Through many years of experience, I can usually tell a person's health and general condition by looking at the person's feet. This is especially true where there are conditions of deformity or extra growth of corns and/or calluses.

These conditions could quite easily be affecting the reflexes in that area, which in turn could affect the organ, gland or part of the body associated with it.

When a Reflexologist notes such conditions as corns or calluses, extra work is needed to help these areas. However, if there is a preponderence of such conditions, it is usually suggested that they be treated by a Podiatrist. It has been my experience that, once the corns and calluses have been removed by a Podiatrist, working this region helps to alleviate the condition and they do not return as easily as before. Many times they do not reappear **at all.**

A note on the particular conditions of corns. It is more difficult working with corns because the area is frequently very sensitive. My recommended method is to work around the area to ease the pain of this condition first, then as I work, it becomes less sensitive and I find that I can work the entire area.

BUNIONS

Inflammation and thickening of the bursa of the joint of the great toe. To work for a bunion, you will hold the great toe with the holding hand, lightly pulling the great toe to straighten it. With the working thumb I will use the basic thumb technique and work all around and then directly on the bunion. This area could be worked on every day. A little self help would be beneficial.

SPURS

While discussing bones of the feet, it might be well to touch upon one particular problem area . . . the calcaneal spur. (**See Figure 5.31**). These are formed by mineral build-up on the end of the calcaneous bone of the heel. The Reflexologist must work the area of a spur with a special zeal.

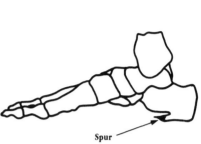

Spur

Figure 5.31

It should be noted that this particular procedure causes some discomfort but is very effective. With spurs, you should schedule regular sessions every day, or at least every other day. Begin by lightly working the area **around** the spur with regular thumb technique. Gradually working up to and on the spur itself, you should gradually increase the pressure during your session.

If you approach the area properly and come in on the area from every direction by using alternate thumbs over the spot and also use a lot of ankle rotating motions, you will help to improve the circulation to that area. This, in turn, helps nature to remove the microscopic waste products and carry them through the bloodstream.

Remember: For best results, this region could be worked every day. This is one of those rare exceptions where it is not necessary to give a full treatment each time you work on this condition.

FOR BROKEN BONES

To review our discussion in **Chapter 2**, where we compare the arm to the leg, etc., it is obvious that we will not work directly on the damaged area for a broken foot, instead,

83

working with the basic thumb and finger technique, we would follow a distinct regimen including:

- for a broken hand, work the corresponding area of the foot.

- for a broken leg, work the corresponding area of the arm at the corresponding site of the break.

- for a broken arm, work the corresponding area of the leg on the same side.

- for a broken finger, work the corresponding area of the toe on the same side.

Once this becomes clear, you should be able to immediately grasp the significance of referral areas. But always remember that it is easier to work the arm for leg problems than it is to work the leg for arm problems. This is primarily due to the heavy muscular structure of the leg making it difficult to reach the reflexes.

In cases of sprain, a trained Reflexologist will immediately work the referral area in order to help stop inflammation and swelling. After the area shows signs of improvement, a light and direct application will serve to improve circulation and thus aid in the healing process.

This chapter is an extremely important one and one which should be read and re-read since the spine, nerves and muscles play such an important part in Reflexology.

DISORDERS OF THE SKELETAL SYSTEM

DISORDER	DESCRIPTION	REFLEX AREAS TO WORK
Ankylosis	Abnormal immobility and fixation of a joint.	Work directly on the area; also referral area (arm or leg) and area on foot.
Arthritis	Ailments involving joints, muscles and tendons. Also called "rheumatism."	All over—entire foot. Work the reflex to the region most affected.
Bunion	Inflammation and thickening of the bursa of the joint of the great toe.	Work around and directly on the bunion.
Bursitis	Inflammation of a bursa. In the patella joint, it is called "housemaid's knee." In the elbow, "tennis elbow." In the shoulder, "bursitis."	Work the reflex to the affected area, the adrenal glands, and the referral area.
Fracture	A crack or break in an arm or a leg.	Work reflex to the affected area on the foot. Work the corresponding referral area in either the arm or leg.
Gout	Acute arthritis and inflammation of a joint.	Work the kidneys and the reflex to the affected area.
Scoliosis	Lateral curvature of the spine.	Reflex to the whole spine, all glands, chest/lung area, shoulder.

DISORDERS OF THE NERVOUS SYSTEM

DISORDER	DESCRIPTION	REFLEX AREAS TO WORK
Bell's Palsy	Paralysis of a facial nerve.	Cervicals, diaphragm.
Encephalitis	Inflammation of the brain and its covering.	Great toes, all toes, all glands.
Epilepsy	A disorder of the nervous system. Major symptom is convulsive seizures.	Diaphragm, colon, ileocecal, whole spine, neck area, all glands.
Headache	One of the most common ailments of man and is a symptom rather than a disorder. Most result from vasodilation of blood vessels in tissues surrounding the brain or from tension in neck or scalp muscles. Stress on whole body.	Whole spine, diaphragm, all glands, all toes.
Hiccoughs	Spasmodic involuntary contractions of the diaphragm that result in un-controlled breathing in of air.	Diaphragm, stomach.
Insomnia	Sleeplessness. An inability to fall asleep easily or to remain asleep.	Diaphragm, all glands.
Meningitis	Inflammation of the meninges that cover the brain and spinal cord.	Great toes, whole spine, all glands.
Multiple Sclerosis	A disease causing hardened patches throughout the brain and spinal cord interfering with nerves in those areas.	Whole spine, all glands, diaphragm.
Parkinson's disease	Disease of the brain causing stiffness of the muscles and characterized by tremors.	Whole spine, all glands, diaphragm, chest/lung area.
Tic douloureux	Trigeminal neuralgia. A painful disorder of the trigeminal nerve characterized by severe pain in the face and forehead.	Neck area, cervicals, diaphragm.

		Whole spine, diaphragm.
Tremors	An involuntary trembling of the body or limbs.	Whole spine, diaphragm.
Vertigo	Dizziness. A sensation of rotation or movement.	Ear reflex, neck area, cervicals, great toes.

DISORDERS OF THE MUSCULAR SYSTEM

DISORDER	DESCRIPTION	REFLEX AREAS TO WORK
Cramps (feet, legs, etc.)	A prolonged spasm and pain in a muscle.	Hip/knee, hip/sciatic, lower spine, parathyroid, adrenals.
Myasthenia gravis	Great muscular weakness without atrophy of the muscles	Adrenal glands, parathyroid.
Ruptured disk	Rupture of a disk, or pad of cartilage between the vertebrae. Sometimes called a "slipped disk."	Work affected areas of spine.
Spasm (see cramps)	A sudden, involuntary contraction of a muscle.	Hip/knee, hip/sciatic, lower spine, parathyroid, adrenals.
Sprain	Excessive stretching of the ligaments of a joint capsule.	Work reflex area on foot; work referral area to affected area.
Strain	Excessive stretching of the ligaments of a joint capsule.	Work reflex area on foot; work referral area to affected area.

For a detailed listing of all disorders, see the charts at the back of this book.

Chapter 6

THE CARDIOVASCULAR SYSTEM

"For the life of the flesh is in the blood . . ."

Leviticus 17:11

THE CARDIOVASCULAR SYSTEM

Pumping vital nutrients and oxygen to all of the tissues of the body and in turn, carrying away their waste products, including carbon dioxide, is the primary task of that magnificent muscle . . . the heart. It causes blood to circulate through a system of arteries, capillaries, and veins.

THE HEART

The heart, the body's most powerful muscle, is a hollow, muscular organ about the size of your clenched fist and it pumps almost 5 liters of blood a minute while you are resting and about 35 liters of blood during exercise.

Putting it another way, the heart's pumping action circulates about 2000 gallons (7570 liters) of blood through an estimated 70,000 miles (112,630 kilometers) of blood vessels every 24 hours.

THE CARDIOVASCULAR SYSTEM (*Figure 6.1*).

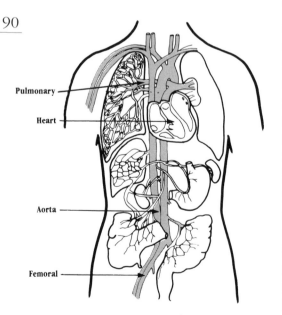

Pulmonary

Heart

Aorta

Femoral

Figure 6.1

The heart is located in an oblique position within the thoracic cavity; one third of it is situated on the right side of the midline while the remaining two thirds are to the left. It is composed of four distinct compartments: the left and right atria and the left and right ventricles. The pumping cycle consists of a contraction (called *systole*) and resting/filling stage (called *diastole*). The right side of the heart receives blood from the veins which has been collected throughout the body and pumps that blood to the lungs to exchange the carbon dioxide waste for fresh oxygen. The left side of the heart receives the oxygen-filled blood and pumps it back into circulation.

This hardest of working muscles must, of course, be enriched and fed with its own blood at all times. (The brain is the only other organ in the human body which actually needs more blood and oxygen than the heart itself). As a matter of fact, it is estimated that the heart keeps about five percent of all of the blood it pumps. This blood is fed into the heart muscle fibers by the coronary arteries which surround the outside of the heart. It is here, in the coronary arteries, where a build up of a certain type of cholesterol in one of these main arteries can stop the flow of blood to the heart muscle, leading to what is called a myocardial infarction: the death of heart muscle tissue . . . we know this situation as a *heart attack*.

LUNG/OXYGEN EXCHANGE

The blood is carried to the lungs by the pulmonary artery. In the lungs, and within the tiny capillaries, the blood trades carbon dioxide for fresh new oxygen. The pulmonary veins then carry the blood back to the left atrium of the heart where it begins its journey to the parts of the body. (*See Figure 6.2*).

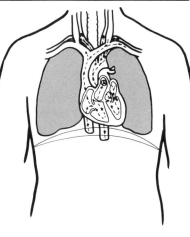

91

Figure 6.2

PULSE

The beat of the heart causes surges of blood through the arteries . . . not in a steady flow, but in waves of pressure. These waves travel through the arteries. When you place your finger over an artery, you can feel the beat or the surge of pressure . . . called the arterial pulse or simply *pulse*.

To the trained Reflexologist whose concern is to keep the bodily systems in balance, the Cardiovascular System is extremely important.

The Reflexologist works these reflexes almost as *second nature,* since this type of preventive therapy can assure the other systems an adequate supply of those nutrients necessary for life. Many circulatory problems are helped by working all the reflexes of the feet.

Elsewhere in this book, I have made mention of the debilitating effects of stress and tension on the human body. This is nowhere more evident than in the cardiovascular system . . . that essential and intricate lifeline to the organs and cells. Stress and tension act as a *tourniquet on this system* since tense muscles tighten over the blood vessels and shut off the supply of nutrients and that ever-so-important oxygen.

Since one of the basic advantages of Reflexology is in the improvement of circulation, you can easily see that working the heart reflex is an excellent preventive measure for heart problems. But, and I cannot stress too often, any reflex area when worked correctly, will automatically improve circulation to that part of the body.

Unfortunately, with the circulatory system there is no *X marks the spot* like the other reflex areas on the foot. And this is a logical conclusion since blood is circulated to all parts of the body. Therefore, you must work all reflex areas of the foot.

And since circulation is only as good as the pump keeping it moving, you should also be aware of the part exercise and diet play in keeping an adjunctive preventive program of Reflexology.

Exercise on a regular basis . . . a brisk walk of a mile or two a day, a climb up several flights of stairs, jumping on a mini-trampoline, or more strenuous activities all help to keep the heart strong and the blood circulating normally.

As far as diet is concerned, most knowledgeable people know that extra pounds mean extra work for the heart.

When you consider that it has been estimated that every pound of excess fat contains about twenty miles of capillaries for blood to be pumped through, you have some small idea of why diet is important to a healthy heart.

Besides the heart itself, and the arteries and veins which play such an important role in this system, there are other vital areas we will be discussing and with which you should become familiar.

Think of the kidneys and how they are affected by high blood pressure. Specifically the liver, the lungs, the portal and renal arteries, all of these must be considered when discussing the cardiovascular system. Now would be a good time to study *Figure 6.3* which delineates this system and related organs.

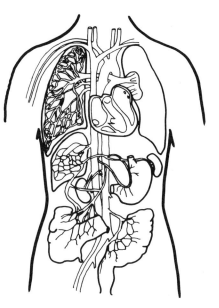

Figure 6.3

You should also be familiar with the following associative heart disease terms:

Angina Pectoris—due to an inadequate supply of blood to the muscle tissue of the heart. Generally, the result of a spasm of the arteries feeding the heart or a clogged condition of these arteries.

Aneurysm—a dilation of the wall of an artery forming a sac—much like a weak spot on an inner tube.

Arrythmia—an abnormally irregular heart beat.

Arteriosclerosis—*Hardening* of the arteries caused by a thickening in the layers of the artery wall. Do not confuse this with . . .

Atherosclerosis—this is one sort of Arteriosclerosis where fatty deposits accumulate in the inside of an artery—much like lime deposits in the pipes of your water system at home.

Coronary Occlusion—an obstruction which interferes with the flow of blood through an artery in the heart. This may result in Angina Pectoris, myocardial infarction or arrythmia. It can be caused by a clot or Arteriosclerosis.

High Blood Pressure—(*Hypertension*)—a continuous elevation in blood pressure. It is the pressure which blood exerts within the blood vessels. Since the heart is a pump, it alternates between contraction and relaxation. The contraction phase is called systole, the relaxation phase is known as diastole. Blood pressure is commonly referred to as two numbers. The *systole* number refers to the pressure of the heart at work; the lower *diastole* number is the pressure while the heart relaxes. The lower figure is the more important one . . . it tells how much your heart is getting to rest. High blood pressure is due primarily to a spasm of the muscles of the arteries, but may also be brought on by arteriosclerosis. Some of the effects of hypertension are: cardiac hypertrophy, with eventual cardiac failure; further hardening of the arteries (*arteriosclerosis*); possible rupture of blood vessels, especially in the brain (*cerebral hemorrhage, "apoplexy"*); kidney dysfunction due to degenerative changes in renal vessels and visual disfunction due to blood vessel change in the eyes or brain. There are two types of arterial hypertension: **primary** or **essential,** in which the hypertension is not preceded by kidney disorder or other pathologic condition, and **renal** hypertension, which accompanies Bright's disease (***nephritis***) and is initiated by renal damage or malfunctioning.

Phlebitis—this is an inflammation of a vein and can be associated with a blood clot within a vein. Usually occurs in lower extremities.

Varicose Veins—swollen, knotted veins usually in the legs. They happen when the walls of the veins become weak and blood cannot be returned properly to the heart. Blood tends to stagnate in the vein and can lead to phlebitis.

Cardiac Arrhythmias—changes in the rhythm of the cardiac contractions caused by disturbances of the electrical activity within the heart muscle.

Coronary Artery Disease (CAD)—a narrowing or occlusion of the coronary arteries or any of their branches.

Myocardial Infarction—damage to a portion of the cardiac muscle as a result of an occlusion of one of the coronary arteries.

Rheumatic Valvular Disease—damage to a heart valve caused by rheumatic fever.

95

WORKING THE CARDIOVASCULAR SYSTEM

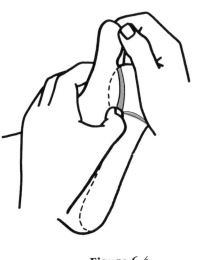

Figure 6.4

The Heart Area—work the heart area across the metatarsals of the left foot above the diaphragm up to the base of the toes. Generally, the most sensitive area is between the first and the second toes (**See Figure 6.4**). Work all the way across the foot to the shoulder reflex area on both the top and the bottom of the foot. You will work the same as described for the lungs. Do not forget the nerve supply going to the heart . . . the vagus nerve as well as many other nerves in that area. Work the cervicals and thoracics as well.

I will also work the area between the first and second zones on the right foot from the diaphragm to the base of the toes, both top and bottom. I always recommend working the left shoulder reflex when I work for heart conditions since many people have some discomfort in the shoulder and arm when they have heart problems.

A good helper area for some heart conditions would be the adrenal glands as adrenaline is often given to people who have heart attacks.

Hypertension—Be sure to work the diaphragm reflex in all cases of hypertension. (**See Chapter 4** for more details on working the diaphragm).

Blood Clots—Nature usually takes care of a blood clot by eventually dissolving or absorbing it. Reflexology can help nature dissolve the clot faster simply by working the referral to the clot area which naturally helps to absorb or dissolve it. We do not work directly on the blood clot itself.

Phlebitis—usually found in the leg; we can work a corresponding area on the arm if the phlebitis is in the leg.

Varicose Veins—I generally recommend working the colon reflex and the corresponding areas of the arm.

Stroke—in a stroke, we know that a blood vessel ruptures or a clot in the brain has already occurred, and the damage has been done. Now we must work the area in order to help the brain repair itself. It is important to remember, if the paralysis is on the **right side of the body,** it indicates damage to the **opposite** hemisphere of the brain . . . therefore, we work the brain area (tip of the great toe) on the left foot (**See Figure 6.5**). This is important to remember when working for a stroke. (**See Chapter 5,** *Nervous System, for working the brain*).

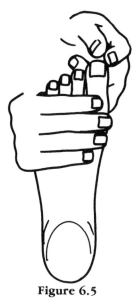

Figure 6.5

Always work the opposite side of the brain:

If stroke is evident on the left side . . . work the tip of the right great toe.

If stroke is evident on the right side . . . work the tip of the left great toe.

DISORDERS OF THE CARDIOVASCULAR SYSTEM

DISORDER	DESCRIPTION	REFLEX AREAS TO WORK
Angina Pectoris	Severe thoracic pain which tends to radiate from the region of the heart to the shoulder and down the left arm. It is accompanied by a feeling of suffocation. It is due to an inadequate supply of blood to the myocardium of the heart, generally the result of coronary spasm or thrombosis.	Heart/lung, cervicals, thoracics, sigmoid colon, diaphragm.
Arteriosclerosis	"Hardening" of the arteries. A condition in which there is thickening and loss of elasticity of the layers of the artery wall. Arteriosclerosis is common in advanced age.	All glands, work entire foot.
Atherosclerosis	A type of arteriosclerosis in which fatty deposits accumulate in the artery.	Thyroid, all glands, work entire foot.
Coronary Occlusion	Obstruction of or interference with the flow of blood through an artery owing to either narrowing of the lumen of the vessels from arteriosclerosis or presence of a thrombus or embolus. The deprivation of oxygen and accumulation of metabolic substances stimulate the pain endings of afferent nerves, giving rise to agonizing chest pains (angina pectoris). Attacks are usually precipitated by muscular exertion or emotional excitement.	same as for angina.
High Cholesterol	May be contributing factor in heart and circulatory diseases, particularly in the formation of fatty deposits in the arteries.	Thyroid, liver.
Hypertension (High Blood Pressure)	A condition in which the blood pressure is persistently *above* that which is normal for a given age level.	Diaphragm; and also kidneys, pituitary, adrenals, thyroid.

Hypotension (Low Blood Pressure)	A condition in which the blood pressure is persistently *below* that which is normal for a given age level.	Adrenals; and also Pituitary, thyroid.
Phlebitis	Inflammation of a vein, usually accompanied by formation of pus. It frequently leads to the formation of thrombus within a vein (thrombophlebitis) which may break loose and result in the distribution of infective emboli to other parts of the body. Phlebitis occurs most commonly in the veins of the lower extremities, often following long confinement in bed, abdominal operations, or childbirth.	Adrenals, colon, liver, referral area: arm.
Stroke	Rupture or blockage of a blood vessel in the brain; results in loss of consciousness, paralysis or other symptoms of brain damage.	Tip of great toe (opposite side from paralysis), other toes, Reflexes to affected areas.
Tachycardia	Excessive rapidity of heart beat. In paroxysmal tachycardia the heart begins suddenly to beat at an abnormally high rate, as fast as 150 or more beats per minute.	Adrenals, heart, cervicals, thoracics, thyroid.
Varicose Veins	Swollen, knotted, and tortuous veins, most commonly seen in the lower extremities. They are brought on by weakening of the walls of the veins or interference with venous return. Blood tends to stagnate in the vessels, and valves become incompetent.	Colon, liver, adrenals, referral area: arm

For a detailed listing of all disorders, see the charts at the back of this book.

Chapter 7

THE LYMPHATIC SYSTEM

*"Know ye not that your body is the temple
of the Holy Spirit, which is in you, which ye
have of God, and ye are not your own?"*

1 Cor. 6–19

THE LYMPHATIC SYSTEM
(*Figure 7.1*)

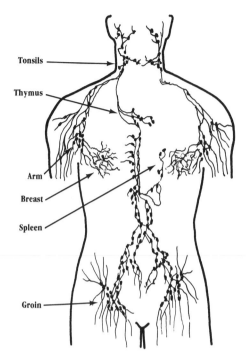

Tonsils

Thymus

Arm

Breast

Spleen

Groin

Figure 7.1

This system's vessels form a network throughout the body almost like the blood vessels, only they contain a high number of valves; the system is usually thought of as being part of the cardiovascular system.

Lymph is derived from the blood plasma and is a colorless fluid rich in cells. As the plasma circulates throughout the body, some of it seeps through the capillary walls as well as from other blood vessels; this leaked fluid is lymph. One of its primary functions is to supply a fluid environment between the cells and the tissues . . . it actually *bathes* them. To keep this fluid circulating, there is a drainage field within the body which ends up in so called collecting stations, or nodes. The lymph carries dead and worn out cells as well as harmful bacteria and viruses along with it to these collecting stations...there are several hundred of these nodes throughout the body. The nodes can be thought of as **outposts** for defense against the harmful bacteria, virus, etc., approaching the interior of the body. Many of us are familiar with the swollen nodes in the groin, breast, neck and armpit...the most notable of these nodes.

THE SPLEEN

The largest mass of lymphatic tissue in the body is the spleen whose main function is the production of protective antibodies. The spleen also acts as a blood filter, since it has the responsibility of ridding the body of old red blood cells and bacteria. Iron storage is another of its functions. This is important since it helps to produce hemoglobin from old cells . . . quite important to the Reflexologist when working on anemia and related dysfunctions.

THE TONSILS

The tonsils are also included in this system since they are composed of masses of lymphoid tissue. The only known function of the tonsils is the formation of antibodies as well as serving as special filters.

THE THYMUS

The thymus is a lymphatic organ located just in front of, and above, the heart. This organ grows rather rapidly from birth to puberty and then begins to diminish in size. As a matter of fact, an adult lives quite comfortably without one. Since it does play an important part in producing antibodies and controlling the body's immune system during childhood, it represents a very important reflex to work in children.

WORKING THE LYMPHATIC SYSTEM

Since the lymphatic system is closely allied with the cardiovascular system, it is not too surprising to learn that every area in which we work on the feet indirectly helps the lymphatic system. This is not to say that the system should be ignored, not in the least. What I am really pointing out is that there are several vital areas which we must always consider when working this system.

GROIN AREA

The first of these key areas is referred to as the groin reflex area. Since the groin is located on the body where the upper leg is joined to the torso, the corresponding reflex area on the foot is where the ankle and the foot meet. This specific reflex area represents the location within the body of a large cluster of lymph nodes and where, often times, there is congestion within these nodes which creates problems for the entire system. Therefore, we must concentrate a great deal of attention and effort on this reflex.

To work the groin reflex area, we must first of all remember to keep the foot in an upward or straight position being sure not to tip it either to the right or to the left or even pull it forward as we work. Pulling the foot forward is often a natural thing since we are trying to see exactly where we are working. It is better to resist that temptation because you will not get into the reflex area in a proper manner.

Now, keeping the foot straight, we place our fingers along the Achilles tendon, the thumbs will be on the bottom of the foot at the waistline and the index fingers of both hands will be on the ankle reflex for the groin. We can then take the fingers of either the right or the left hand (*we will be using both*) and we then walk them in a forward motion, first one and then the other, lifting them to come back and to start the walk again (***See Figure 7.2***). We work this region several times in this manner with both fingers. You will notice that the fingers get into the reflex area a lot easier. I also prefer to use my fingers in order not to tire the thumb which will be used for the more difficult tasks. That is not to say you cannot use the thumb if you happen to find it easier and more convenient. Just make sure to work all around the area where the ankle is joined to the foot and then work in both directions.

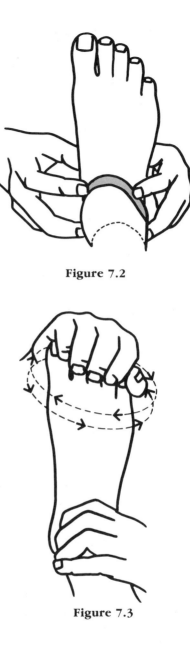

Figure 7.2

There is also a relaxing technique which is appropriate to use here. Place the hand with fingers together over the top of the foot with the webbing between the thumb and fingers over the ankle joint (groin area). The rest of the fingers are firmly wrapped around the leg. Then we take the other hand and we do the ankle rotation . . . rotating the foot several times in one direction and then several times in the opposite direction (*See Figure 7.3*).

105

Figure 7.3

This too, can be done with either hand. Of course, one hand may seem a little easier for you than the other, but remember that this process can and should be repeated on both feet. This is very important!

CHEST, LUNG, BREAST AREA

The next important area in discussing the lymphatic system is the lungs, chest and breast reflex.

We know that there exists rather large lymph networks in the breast and in the arm pits, so this region is very important to the Reflexologist. This particular reflex is located from the diaphragm guideline to the base of the toes . . . from the small toe to the great toe on both the top and the bottom of both feet.

I have found that it is much easier to work these reflexes on the top of the foot since the heavy padding on the bottom of the foot makes it difficult to work. This, of course, does not mean that we cannot work the bottom of the foot, but experience has indicated that the top of the foot is much more effective in working this specific reflex.

This particular region will be worked using the fingers on the top part of each foot; the thumb is the only method for working the bottom. We will use both hands remembering to keep the foot in an upright position. Again, I must advise you **not** to pull the foot towards you just so you can see the area you are working.

We can either start working from the little toe side or the great toe side of the foot. It is important to work across the foot in both directions using both hands separately. This enables us to contact both sides of the metatarsal grooves.

Actually, when we work between the first and second toe just below the base of the toe we will be working what we refer to as the lymph drainage area. This represents the area where the thoracic duct and the drainage for the lymphatic system are located. Anatomically, it is where the subclavian and the jugular veins come together deep in the base of the neck on both sides . . . so naturally, this is the reflex area for lymphatic drainage.

In all cases, this region across the top of the foot representing the lung, chest and breast, is extremely helpful for the lymphatics.

Another important area to work is the shoulder reflex since many lymph nodes are located in that region. (The detailed discussion on working this reflex area will be discussed in *Chapter 9*).

TONSILS AND ADENOIDS

An additional and rather important area of the lymphatic system is the tonsil/adenoid reflex. These reflexes will be located on the great toe since that is the reflex to our neck and head. Be sure to work the neck reflex and **not** that area where the toe is joined onto the foot. The tonsil/adenoid reflex will be located around the great toe region approximately one-third from the base of the toes. Anatomically, we know that the tonsils are located in the upper region of the neck, consequently, the reflex will be approximately one-third of the way up the toe from the base.

Let the index finger work around from the inside edge to the outside edge on the top of the great toe. The right thumb will work from the inside edge to the outside edge on the bottom of the toe. We can then come back on both the top and the bottom in the opposite direction with the alternate thumb and finger. This reflex will be found on both feet.

The helper area for the tonsils and adenoids will be the small toes.

(One thing to remember: when we work the toes, they **are** small and usually require that we change hands and attempt to work them in both directions with each thumb. As I have stated, there are many reflexes which require our approaching them at different angles in order to find them. It is not always the same angle with this reflex region as it is with some of the others in which we have specific points to find.)

THYMUS

Another part of the lymphatic system is the thymus which is located below the thyroid in the sternum (breastbone). This reflex is located below the thyroid reflex and alongside of the upper thoracics. The region which we describe on the chart as relative to the thyroid is also an excellent area for the thymus.

We work this reflex area with our basic thumb technique from the diaphragm reflex to the base of the toes in the whole first zone. This reflex is important for children.

Now, let's take a specific look at some particular dysfunctions and corresponding reflex areas to work.

DISORDERS OF THE LYMPHATIC SYSTEM

DISORDER	DESCRIPTION	REFLEX AREAS TO WORK
Ankles (swollen)	The presence of abnormally large amounts of fluid in the tissue spaces around the ankles.	Kidneys, Adrenals, Lymph System; Referral Area: Wrist.
Breast Lumps	Most lumps of the breasts are benign and are usually infected lymph nodes.	Chest/Lung, Lymph System, Pituitary.
Edema	The presence of abnormally large amounts of fluid in the intercellular tissue spaces of the body.	Lymph System, Kidneys, Adrenals.
Fluid Retention	Same as edema.	Lymph System, Kidneys, Adrenals
Infections	An invasion of the body by bacteria.	Adrenals, Lymph System, Region or Area Affected.
Leukemia	A disease of the blood-forming organs, characterized by an increase in the number of leukocytes and their precursors in the blood, causing enlargement and proliferation of the lymphoid tissue of the spleen, lymphatic glands, and bone marrow.	All Glands, Lymph System, Spleen.
Sore Throat	Inflammation of the throat and tonsils.	Lymph System, All Toes, Great Toes, Adrenals, Cervicals.
Tonsillitis	Inflammation of the tonsil, a small mass of lymphoid tissue.	Great Toes, Lymph System, All Toes, Adrenals, Cervicals.

For a detailed listing of all disorders, see the charts at the back of this book.

Chapter 8

THE SENSE ORGANS

" . . . For I am fearfully and wonderfully made . . ."

Psalms 139:14

THE SENSE ORGANS

This special system includes those sense organs which are used to make the body aware of its environment both outside and inside of the body. (**See Figure 8.1**)

These sense organs will include:

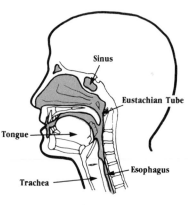

Figure 8.1

- **The Skin**—*Touch*

- **The Eyes**—*Vision*

- **The Ears**—*Hearing and Equilibrium*

- **The Nose**—*Smell*

- **The Tongue**—*Taste*

These sense organs are commonly classified according to the type of information the body receives.

- There are sensations which give information about the external environment. They include touch, pressure, temperature, pain, hearing, sight and smell.

- The sense organs which give information about the internal environment. They include pain, taste, fatigue, hunger, thirst, nausea, etc.

- The sense organs which give information about the body's position and movement . . . the sense of equilibrium . . . the inner ear.

THE SKIN AS A SENSE ORGAN

The skin is much more than just a *wrapper* keeping the body together. It produces at least one important vitamin "D." It is also responsible for helping to regulate body temperature through a complex *thermostat*. The skin is also the barrier which bacteria must penetrate before causing damage to the organs and systems of the body. The skin contains the millions of sweat glands which help to regulate the body's temperature as well as keep the delicate balance between salt and water. The skin is an important excretory organ serving in the healthy person to excrete about 500 c.c.'s of water as it regulates body temperature. The complex structure of the network of nerves within the skin is awesome . . . many of which act as receptor organs for the sense of touch and pain, as well as cold and heat.

The Olfactory Sense—*(sense of smell)*. The nose is an organ which not only is used for the sense of smell, but is also used to *clean* and condition the air before it enters the lungs . . . warming the air on a cold day, freeing it of particles and irritants and giving it the proper moisture. The nose is capable of recognizing 4,000 different scents through the utilization of special receptor cells on the roof of each nasal cavity.

The Gustatory Sense—*(sensations of taste)*. Taste is accomplished through the use of receptors or *taste buds* on the tongue itself. The tongue not only aids in the sensation of taste, but it is also essential to speech and to aid in swallowing food. But taste is of primary importance to the tongue which automatically recognizes four primary groups: sour, salty, bitter and sweet. Sweet taste buds are located mainly on the tip of the tongue, bitter at the back, salty at the sides and tip, and sour at the sides.

The Visual Sense—The visual organ of sight, the eye, is perhaps one of the most complex organs in the body. Millions of nerve connections can handle over a million simultaneous messages. When looking at a cut-away drawing of the eye, you can easily compare it to a camera. The *window* of the eye, the cornea actually bends the light rays; the pupil which is an adjustable *iris* allows only the right amount of light to enter. The lens adjusts the focus by a series of muscles which flatten it for distance vision and

113

allow it to fatten for near vision. The lens is surrounded by fluid. Light passing through the fluid and the lens is focused on the retina which covers most of the interior of the eye. Millions of light sensitive receptor cells are contained in the retina . . . some shaped like rods, for black and white vision, others are cones for sharp color vision. All impulses received at the retina are carried to the brain through the optic nerve.

SPECIFIC DISORDERS OF THE EYE INCLUDE:

Myopia, or nearsightedness, a condition in which light rays come to a focus slightly in front of the retina.

Hyperopia, a farsightedness, a condition in which the light rays come to a focus slightly behind the retina.

Astigmatism due to irregularities in the curvature of the cornea or of the lens.

Cataract is a loss of transparency of the crystalline lens.

Glaucoma is caused when intraocular pressure increases because of an overproduction of intraocular fluid or because the drainage canal becomes blocked.

Tunnel Vision is when the field of vision becomes narrowed.

Conjunctivitis is an inflammation of the membrane which lines the eyelids.

Detached Retina is a complete or partial separation of the retina from the inner layers of the eye (choroid).

Sties are a bacterial infection of one of the sebaceous glands of the eyelid.

HEARING AND EQUILIBRIUM

The ear is a complex organ, not only of hearing, but also of balance. It is divided into 1) the external ear, 2) the middle ear, and 3) the inner ear. (*See Figure 8.2*).

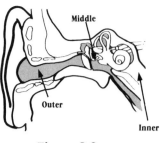

Figure 8.2

The outer ear gathers sound much like a disk antenna one sees scanning the skies during an orbital flight. It picks up the sound, sends it down the one-inch canal to the ear drum or tympanic membrane. The ear drum is set in motion by the sound waves hitting it. This vibratory motion is magnified about 22 times its original force through a series of three small bones called the anvil, hammer and stirrup (since they actually resemble an *anvil*, *hammer* and *stirrup*). From here, the sound goes to the inner ear.

The inner ear is made up of a complicated series of canals which contain sensory receptors. The main component is called the cochlea because it looks like a snail's shell; it is made up of a spiral canal which is filled with microscopic nerve cells . . . each one *pre-tuned* to a particular vibration. When a nerve cell (actually very thin hair cells) vibrate, it produces a minute electrical current which goes into the acoustic nerve . . . the nerve of hearing, called the auditory nerve. This particular nerve sends the impulse to the brain for translation.

115

The inner ear has another very important function to perform . . . that of equilibrium or *balance*. This is accomplished by a unique arrangement of structures called the semi-circular ducts filled with a fluid called endolymph. One of the canals reads up and down motion, one forward motion, and the third one lateral or side motion.

Motion of the body causes the fluid in one of the canals to be displaced and tiny hair cells detect the fact and send it to the brain which orders the body to *get back in balance*.

Pressure within the middle ear cavity is equalized with external pressure through the Eustachian tube. The Eustachian tube runs from the middle ear to the pharynx and provides an air passage which equalizes pressure on both sides of the eardrum. The middle ear is often the site of infection, particularly in children. This infection of the middle ear is called Otitis Media and can lead to serious difficulties. The middle ear is directly connected with the mastoid air cells contained in the mastoid bone just behind the outer ears.

WORKING THE SENSE ORGANS

EYE AND EAR REFLEX

These important reflexes are located in the same area on both feet . . . at the base of the small toes (**See Figure 8.3**).

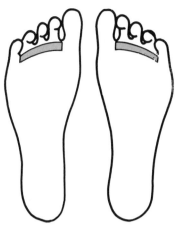

When working this reflex area, we will alternate our right hand with the left hand.

The eye and ear reflex is a rather difficult one in that the technique I recommend is a bit different from those used for other reflex areas.

Figure 8.3

I usually start on the right foot with the right hand as the working hand. The fingers of the left hand (holding hand) are placed on top of the foot at the base of the small toes.

The thumb is placed on the padding of the metatarsal and gently pulls the padding down toward the heel. I always stress the word *gently* because you should never exert excessive pressure in this maneuver. Note how the thumb is flat against the

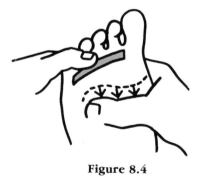

Figure 8.4

metatarsal area along the bottom of the foot. (**See Figure 8.4**).

Place the right thumb of the working hand on the ridge making sure to use the **outside** edge of the thumb. **(Chapter 4)** The ridge is formed where the base of the small toes meet the metatarsal padding. I have coined the phrase *walking the ridge* especially for this maneuver since it seems to adequately describe the working regimen. The thumb will walk in a forward motion across this ridge. I must stress the use of the **outside** edge of the thumb because using the inside edge is less effective. (**See Figure 8.5**).

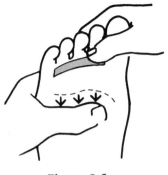

I generally go over this area several times in one direction. Then I will change hands so that the holding hand now becomes the working hand. The holding hand will assume the same position on the toes as previously discussed.

Figure 8.5

The walking motion must be one in which the thumb walks all the way across the base of the small toes, is picked up, comes back and starts over . . . with the pressure of the thumb exerted downward toward the heel.

To gain maximum effectiveness, I recommend a continuous walking with one hand, repeating several times, then changing hands and walking in the opposite direction several times. Repeat this process on the left foot, starting with the left thumb.

Several important things I would particularly like you to notice when working the eye and ear reflex:

- When pulling the padding down with the holding hand, particularly on a heavy *fleshy*, or callused foot, you have to apply a greater degree of pressure downward with the thumb . . . but be very careful that you don't squeeze the area. This causes the padding to push up toward the base of the toes and you will have a difficult time finding the reflex area. Be careful of any broken skin between the toes.

- After working over the area several times, you may frequently notice that working in one direction may be more effective than another for contacting a sensitive reflex point. When you find this spot, you can use the index finger and work straight into the area with the finger tip pointed toward the base of the toe. A slight rotation motion with the finger on this sensitive area is often quite effective. (**See Figure 8.6**).

I would also like to reiterate here that the eye and ear reflexes actually overlap one another. Remember, the "packed suitcase" analogy I made in **Chapter 2**, the ear anatomically lies behind the eye. Frequently, I am asked why we don't just work the great toes for the eye and ear reflexes since they have all five zones in each. The answer to that is based upon years of experience in that it is extremely difficult to find these reflexes in the great toe since they

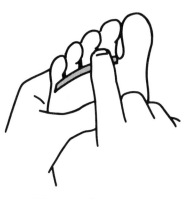

Figure 8.6

would be comparatively smaller. Consequently, I have found that the best results can be obtained by working the base of the toes, as I have outlined.

HELPER AREAS FOR THE EYES AND EARS

Now, I would like to discuss some valuable helper areas for the eye and ear reflex.

The side of the neck reflexes can be found on the outside edge of the great toes (**See Figure 8.7**). Working this area all the way from the tip of the great toe to the base is very important for helping the nerve supply to the eyes and the ears.

Another effective helper area I have found to be effective is the throat region where the great toes are joined onto the feet. This region includes the area between the base of the toe and the "ball" of the toe. This area can be effective for such maladies as ear problems, (ear infections), enlarged tonsils, sluggish lymph glands, and mastoids. This is also the reflex for the eustachian tube.

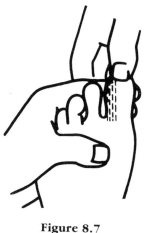

Figure 8.7

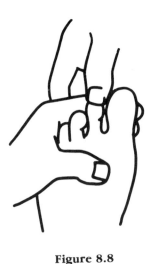

Figure 8.8

Be sure, when working these helper areas, that you do not try to pinpoint a small section, rather work the entire region from where the toe is joined to the foot right up to the first joint of the great toe and around the toe itself.

As a matter of fact, I have found that, because of the zone lines, working all the toes is very helpful for many eye-problems as well as the sinuses. They also often affect one another. (**See Figure 8.8**).

Ears can also be helped by working these same areas since they are in the same zones.

Another helper area for the eyes is the kidney reflex. The kidneys are in the third zone in the body, the same zone as the eyes. Now, we know that there is no anatomical connection between the eye and the kidney, but do you remember grandmother saying, *"dark circles under the eyes indicate kidney problems"*?

Well, through my many years with Reflexology, I can appreciate that old saying, for I have found that working the kidney reflex often is very helpful for some eye problems.

By working the eye reflexes I won't promise that you are going to be able to throw your eye glasses away! What I am saying is that if the eyes are growing weaker, you may be able to prevent further deterioration and not have to change your eye glasses as often.

SKIN REFLEXES

We are surrounded by skin! Everything we do, every reflex we work can help some part of our skin. Every organ, every gland, has some indirect effect on our skin.

But I have found that some glands are key reflex areas for skin conditions ... the endocrines, the thyroid and the adrenals. These are important for such skin conditions as dryness, eczema, psoriasis, hives, and some nerve-related cases of shingles.

The kidneys (*master chemists of the body*) and the liver help to purify the blood and can also have a lot to do with skin conditions. Diet also has a great effect on the skin.

SMELL AND TASTE

The sense organs of smell and taste are naturally located in the middle of the head region so we concentrate on working the middle third of the great toe. (*See Figures 8.9, 8.10*).

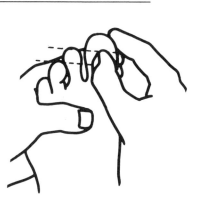

To work this region, we use standard thumb and finger techniques in all directions, up, down and across.

Let me interject a personal view here.

Figure 8.9

In my many travels and in all my seminars, I take the time to preach a small sermon against smoking. The Surgeon General has said it all many times so I only join my small voice with those of the physicians and non-smokers in all areas of the world.

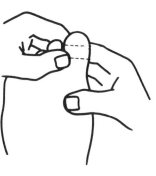

Smoking is destructive . . . it is a habit that can kill you!

Figure 8.10

As a Reflexologist interested in restoring balance and consequent health, you are going to become acquainted with the effects of smoking.

Smoking destroys smell and taste. People who have stopped this habit almost immediately notice how much better their food tastes . . . and they instinctively realize that their sense of smell improves. Nicotine constricts arteries, raises blood pressure, and stimulates the heart to beat harder and faster. Tobacco contains toxic chemicals such as cadmium, radioactive elements, insecticides, and tars. Smokers have a much increased incidence of heart disease and lung cancer compared to their non-smoking counterparts.

But . . . why people who want good health continue to puff away is a mystery to me. You should take every opportunity to dissuade your clients from smoking.

In all likelihood, the addictive nature of smoking explains its hold on so many. Chronic cigarette smoking is a good example of drug dependence. Reduction of tension through Reflexology can assist an individual in breaking this pernicious habit.

My sermon is over. I can only reiterate that working around the area of the great toe is very helpful for taste and smell. This is a natural conclusion when we realize that the taste buds are in the tongue area. The mouth and nose reflexes are found in the middle one-third of the great toe.

The nose, of course, is the organ of smell and also can be the source of discomfort in the form of polyps. The sinuses are helpful to our sense of smell and are also the site of infection. See **Chapter 9** for working the sinuses.

All of these conditions are alleviated by working the entire great toe, throat and head reflex areas as well as all the toes.

The following chart should be studied for detailed approaches to problems of the senses.

DISORDERS OF THE SENSE ORGANS

DISORDER	DESCRIPTION	REFLEX AREAS TO WORK
Acne	A disorder characterized by eruptions or pustules, usually occuring at beginning stages of adulthood.	Liver, adrenals, all glands, kidneys, intestines, thyroid, diaphragm.
Dry Skin		Thyroid, adrenals.
Eczema	A skin rash characterized by itching, swelling, blistering and scaling of skin.	Liver, adrenals, all glands, kidneys, intestines, thyroid, diaphragm.
Halitosis	Offensive breath; bad breath.	Stomach, liver, intestines, great toes.
Lupus	Tuberculosis of the skin marked by formation of reddish brown eruptions.	All glands, intestines, liver, whole spine.
Nose		Great toes, all toes.
Perspiring hands and feet		All glands, liver, intestines, kidneys, diaphragm.
Psoriasis	A chronic skin disease marked by red patches covered with silver scales. Cause unknown.	Thyroid, adrenals, liver, diaphragm, kidneys, intestines, all glands.
Shingles	An acute virus disease characterized by inflamation of spinal ganglia with eruptions along the affected sensory nerve.	Diaphragm, all glands, whole spine.
Tongue		Great toes.

DISORDERS OF THE SENSE ORGANS—EYE

DISORDER	DESCRIPTION	REFLEX AREAS TO WORK
Cataracts	An opacity of the crystalline eye lens.	Eye reflex, neck area, cervicals, all toes, pituitary, kidneys.
Glaucoma	A condition of the eye characterized by increased intraocular pressure	Eye reflex, throat/neck, all toes, kidneys, diaphragm.
Pink Eye	An inflammation of the conjunctiva—contagious.	Eye reflex, all toes, neck, kidneys.
Sty	Inflammation of one or more sebaceous glands of the eyelid.	Eye reflex, neck area, all toes.

DISORDERS OF THE SENSE ORGANS—EAR

DISORDER	DESCRIPTION	REFLEX AREAS TO WORK
Deafness	Complete or partial loss of ability to hear.	Ear reflex, cervicals, side of neck, great toes.
Dizziness	Vertigo. A sensation of unsteadiness with a feeling of movement within the head.	Side of neck, ear reflex, cervicals.
Earache	Inflamed condition of the ear.	Ear reflex, all toes, throat/neck (eustachian tube).
Motion Sickness	Nausea, vomiting, and vertigo induced by irregular or rhythmic movements.	Ear reflex, diaphragm, neck, spine.
Tinnitus	A ringing or tinkling sound in the ear.	Ear reflex, cervicals, neck, great toes.
Vertigo	Balance disturbance, difficulty in maintaining balance.	Ear reflex, neck, cervicals, great toes.

For a detailed listing of all disorders, see the charts at the back of this book.

Chapter 9

THE RESPIRATORY SYSTEM

"The spirit of God hath made me, and the breath of the Almighty hath given me life."

Job 33:4

THE RESPIRATORY SYSTEM

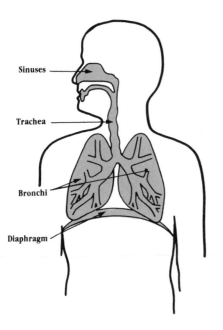

Sinuses

Trachea

Bronchi

Diaphragm

Figure 9.1

The Respiratory System is usually associated with: the nose, the throat region (the pharynx and the larynx), the windpipe (trachea), the bronchi, the sinuses, the lungs, and the diaphragm. (*See Figure 9.1*).

When we think of the Respiratory System, we are concerning ourselves with the exchange of oxygen and carbon dioxide . . . a life-sustaining process we term *breathing*. It's not such a simple operation once you examine the mechanics of breathing more closely.

Adjacent to the nasal cavity are air spaces which are called the paranasal sinuses. They contain mucous glands and have cilia which convey the mucus through small channels into the nasal cavity. These sinuses are important particularly in persons suffering from colds, flu and related illnesses and should not be passed over in working the reflexes associated with the respiratory system. Sinuses are not developed fully until adult life. The younger the child the less the sinuses. Air is inhaled through the nose, pharynx, larynx, trachea, right and left bronchi and finally into the alveoli or air sacs in the lung. It is here that the oxygen is exchanged for the waste material, carbon dioxide.

The trachea branches at the back of the throat (pharynx). The top half of the trachea is the larynx or voice box containing the vocal cords. Below this area, the trachea descends to just behind the sternum and begins to branch into thousands of bronchi, bronchioles and alveoli. The trachea also branches into the right and the left lungs. Both of the lungs are covered by a thin tissue called the pleura

128

which also lines the inside of the thoracic cavity. The large right lung has three distinct lobes: the left lung has only an upper and lower lobe.

The air reaches its final destination in the lungs through the action of the diaphragm. When the diaphragm contracts, it causes the chest cavity to expand, since the chest cavity is a vacuum, and the lungs hang in this cavity, the enlargement of the vacuum area causes air to be drawn into the lungs. When the diaphragm relaxes, the chest walls return to their original position, thus increasing the pressure, which, in turn, forces the air out of the lungs.

Of particular importance to the Reflexologist are the lungs themselves. Each lung is cone-shaped with its base resting on the diaphragm. The tip of each lung (the apex) extends up into the base of the neck. The entire thoracic cavity is lined with a membrane which completely covers the lungs . . . the pleura. When this membrane is inflamed, pleurisy is present.

Several large structures either enter or leave the lungs, including the bronchi, the pulmonary artery and veins, the bronchial arteries and veins and lymphatic vessels.

Let's examine these structures and their functions more closely . . .

The right half of the heart receives the oxygen-poor blood from the veins of the body. This blood enters the heart at the right atrium and then flows down to the right ventricle which pumps the blood to the lungs via the pulmonary artery. In the lungs, the blood passes through tiny capillaries where it picks up oxygen from the alveoli in a chemical *trade off*. This oxygen poor blood carries the carbon dioxide from the cells in the body and *trades* it for oxygen.

In the lungs, the tiny capillaries touch equally small structures called alveoli . . . the smallest air sacs of the lungs. Every breath of air which we take goes into the lungs to fill these air sacs. As a matter of fact, it has been estimated that there are anywhere from 300 million to one billion of these air sacs within our lungs. It is here that the important exchange takes place . . . carbon dioxide for oxygen through the one cell thin walls of the capillaries and the alveoli. The carbon dioxide is then expelled (exhaled) from the body while the oxygen is carried in the blood via veins leading away from the lungs to the left atrium of the heart.

It is estimated that the total surface area within our lungs which is exposed to air is about 600 square feet.

SMOKING AND THE LUNGS

The body's air cleaning process begins with the small hairs in the nose, throat and bronchial passages . . . tiny hairs, called cilia, wave back and forth to trap tiny alien particles. What is important to remember here is that cigarette smoking paralyzes this action. Sometimes these cilia, when constantly exposed to cigarette smoke, die. As a result of faulty ciliary function, particles, mucus and other fluids formed within the air passages often find their way into the alveoli . . . those all-important air sacs. When these sacs become plugged, air cannot be exchanged. The heavy cigarette smoker is in danger of actually drowning as in the case of emphysema.

WORKING THE RESPIRATORY SYSTEM

Working this system is basically working those areas associated with breathing: the lung and chest areas. Actually, some of the reflexes we described in the lymphatic system are almost the same as those for the respiratory system because the breast, chest and lung are in the same area.

LUNGS

As we think of the lungs, the reflex area is located from the diaphragm guideline up to the base of the toes and across the entire foot (from inside to outside) on both top and bottom of the foot as this is our entire lung region.

First, I will work the bottom of the foot; this area is more callused and will need more firmness. When working the area on the bottom of the right foot for the lung reflex area, I place the heel of my left holding hand on the metatarsal padding with the fingers gently over the toes. I tilt the foot slightly outwards and gently spread the toes. Using my right thumb with the basic thumb technique, I will work up the grooves formed by the bones between each toe (**See Figure 9.2**), starting with the groove between the great toe and the second toe ... remember to separate the great toe and the second toe with the holding hand in order to properly open the grooves. After several passes up this area, proceed

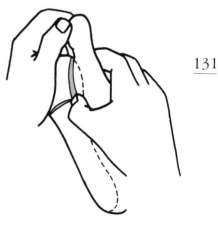

Figure 9.2

with the same technique in the grooves between the second and the third toes; then the third and fourth toes; and then the fourth and fifth toes. I will then change hands and with my left thumb, I will work back in the other direction starting with the groove between the fourth and fifth toes. I repeat this procedure on the left foot, starting with my left thumb.

I also work this same area on the top of the foot. This area usually is very tender and should be worked very gently at first . . . working just to the person's discomfort tolerance.

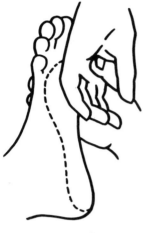

Figure 9.3

I begin with the right foot and use my right hand as my working hand. Placing my left fist on the metatarsal padding, I will push forward to spread the top of the foot. I place the thumb of my right hand inside the fist for leverage and then work down the top of the foot with the inside corner of my index finger (**See Figure 9.3**). I work in the groove between the great toe and the second toe, making sure the fist is pushing as this will spread the region while I am working. I work this area several times and then move to the following grooves repeating this procedure with each groove. Change hands and repeat this procedure in the opposite direction.

Another way to work on the top of the right foot is to use the holding hand (left hand) to spread the great toe and the second toe. Be sure to hold the foot up straight . . . do not pull it forward to see where you are working. The working hand (right hand) will have the thumb placed on the bottom of the foot in the metatarsal padding, pushing forward to spread the area you will be working. The index finger will do the walking in a forward direction on the top of the foot (**See Figure 9.4**). After several passes in this groove, move on to the next groove. Work in this manner all the way to the last groove, between the fourth and fifth toes. Change hands and repeat the procedure in the opposite direction. Be sure not to pull the foot toward you as this will tighten the surface of the foot and thus prevent you from contacting the reflexes.

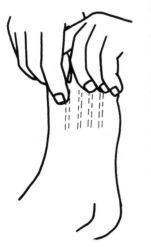

Figure 9.4

132

BRONCHIAL TUBES

When you are working the area between the great toe and second toe, both top and bottom, you will be working the bronchial tubes that lead to the lungs. Remember this area for the chest-lung area is found from the diaphragm guideline to the base of the toes, both top and bottom.

DIAPHRAGM

The diaphragm is a part of the respiratory system since it is an intricate part of our breathing apparatus as well as being a key reflex for tension and stress. The diaphragm is also a reflex where we will find relief for a lot of lung conditions, including pneumonia, bronchitis, asthma, and emphysema. (*See Chapter 4* for working the diaphragm.)

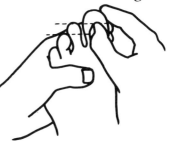

Figure 9.5

NOSE AND THROAT

The reflex to the nose will be found in the middle third of the ball of the great toe (*See Figures 9.5, 9.6*). The nose reflex may be helpful for polyps in the nose as well as for adenoids. The throat reflex area will be found on the neck of the great toe. This reflex is helpful for sore throats, tonsillitis and eustachian tube problems. (For a detailed analysis of working this reflex, see the Sense Organ **Chapter 8**).

133

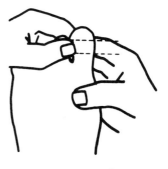

Figure 9.6

SINUSES

The sinus reflexes are found in all of the toes; the great toe having all five zones in it represents the entire head while the four minor toes on each foot are actually used for *fine tuning*.

When working this reflex, we must always remember to support and protect the toes at all times. This is important since the toes are sensitive and the most difficult reflex area to work and master properly.

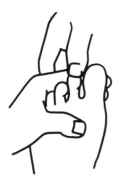

Figure 9.7

Starting on the right foot, we will use the right hand as the working hand and the left as the supporting hand. Place the fingers of the supporting hand horizontal to the toes, with the index finger level with the tip of the toes (*See Figure 9.7*). Place the fingers of the working hand over the outside of the supporting fingers; the first two fingers of the working hand should be over the two knuckles of the supporting fingers (*See Figure 9.8*). Using the basic thumb technique and starting with the great toe, work down the center and then down the outside edge of each toe from its tip to its base. The working hand and the holding hand move together as a unit as you move from toe to toe. Remember, the first fingers of the working hand should be over the two knuckles of the supporting fingers. Be sure to work each toe several times.

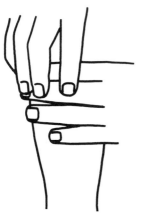

Figure 9.8

134

Then, you change hands and repeat this process with the left thumb, starting on the small toe. Always work **down** the middle and then the inside edge of each toe to its base, remembering that the right hand will be supporting and protecting the toes.

This process is repeated on the left foot with alternate hands. Start with the left hand on the left foot.

Several things to remember when working the sinus reflexes:

- These reflexes generally are quite sensitive, especially the 3rd and 4th toe, so ease up the pressure a bit when working these reflex areas.

- We generally start to work from the tip of the toe to the base; if the toes are long, you **can** work from the base **upward**.

- These reflexes are for anything in the corresponding zone of the head, including eyes, ears and teeth.

- Helper areas include the ileocecal valve, pituitary and adrenals.

The Respiratory System is important to the Reflexologist since many respiratory diseases and associative problems will become familiar to you in your work. Study the following chart carefully.

135

DISORDERS OF THE RESPIRATORY SYSTEM

DISORDER	DESCRIPTION	REFLEX AREAS TO WORK
Adenoids	The so called "pharyngeal tonsils" located in the posterior portion of the nasal cavity. When enlarged, they may obstruct breathing.	Great toes, pituitary.
Asthma	Spasms of the muscles in the bronchial tubes and often an excess secretion of mucus which obstructs the breathing passageways.	Chest/lung, adrenals, ileocecal, diaphragm
Croup	Most often occuring in children, it is a laryngeal spasm which makes breathing very difficult.	Diaphragm, bronchials, ileocecal, chest/lung, all toes.
Emphysema	A condition where the alveoli and the bronchial tubes become over distended by gas or air.	Adrenals, ileocecal, diaphragm, chest/lung, lymph system.
Hay Fever	An allergic disease affecting the mucous membranes of the nose and other respiratory passageways to the conjunctiva of the eyes.	Ileocecal, all toes, all glands, colon, chest/lung.
Pleurisy	Inflammation of the pleura, the membrane lining the thoracic cavity and covering the lungs.	Lymph system, adrenals, diaphragm, chest/lung (top and bottom).
Pneumonia	Inflammation of the lungs caused primarily by bacteria and viruses.	Chest/lung, diaphragm, intestines, all glands, lymph system.
Sinusitis	Inflammation of the sinuses.	All toes, ileocecal, adrenals, chest/lung.
Tonsillitis	Inflammation of the tonsils; also called "quinsy".	Great toes, all toes, lymph system, adrenals, cervicals.

For a detailed listing of all disorders, see charts at the back of this book.

Chapter 10

THE DIGESTIVE SYSTEM

"The fruit thereof shall be for food, and the leaf shall be for medicine."

Ezekiel 47:12

THE DIGESTIVE SYSTEM

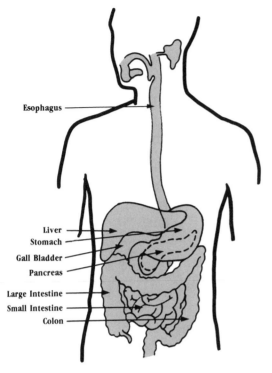

Esophagus

Liver
Stomach
Gall Bladder
Pancreas

Large Intestine
Small Intestine
Colon

Figure 10.1

While the spine is described as the hollow bony structure containing nerves which run to all parts of the body, the digestive system is comprised of a tube . . . the alimentary canal, plus a number of accessory organs. (*See Figure 10.1*)

What is meant by digestion? Simply the process by which certain organs act on ingested food both mechanically and chemically so it can be absorbed and thereby provide nutrition for the body.

Digestion is a process which starts in the mouth with the chewing and mixing of food with saliva containing enzymes. From this point on, the mixture enters the alimentary canal whereupon food is reduced to soluble, absorbable substances. The usable material is absorbed into the body and the waste material eliminated.

The alimentary canal is formed by the mouth, pharynx, esophagus, stomach, small intestine, colon (or large intestine) and rectum.

The accessory organs commonly associated with the digestive system include the salivary glands, liver, gall bladder and pancreas.

The mouth's primary function in digestion is largely mechanical since the food is broken up by the teeth, ground into small particles and moistened by saliva.

The pharynx serves to pass food from the mouth to the esophagus.

The esophagus conveys food from the pharynx to the stomach—passing through the thorax and then through the esophageal hiatus of the diaphragm.

In the stomach, vigorous activity takes place to chemically change the food substances into a more absorbable state.

As food enters the stomach, wave-like contractions sweep from top to bottom so as to mix the food with gastric juices. Located deep within the folds of the stomach's interior are over 35 million glands which secrete up to 3 quarts (2.8 liters) of gastric juices per day. These juices contain hydrochloric acid and pepsin as well as other powerful enzymes needed to break down heavy proteins and other food substances.

The pepsin breaks down the proteins; other juices reduce the food to a semi-liquid consistency called chyme. The amount of time it takes for the stomach to break down food substances varies with the types of food eaten, usually from 3 to 5 hours.

Approximately 85% of the stomach is located on the left side of the body and has a capacity of about two quarts (1.89 liters).

The muscular contractions or peristalsis of the stomach churn the food with the enzymes and work it toward the pyloric valve and into the duodenum, (the beginning of the small intestine).

NOTE: If the stomach acid is not appropriately neutralized in the duodenum area, the acid can irritate the lining which results in an ulcer, a duodenal ulcer. If the ulcer is in the stomach, it is termed a gastric ulcer.

The small intestine plays the major part in digestion and absorption of the nutrients from the food. It is divided into three sections: the duodenum, the jejunum and the ileum. It is important to note that the bile and pancreatic ducts open into the duodenum. Bile and pancreatic juice are important aids to digestion. They also neutralize the acid from the stomach.

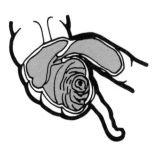

Figure 10.2

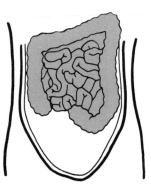

Figure 10.3

The Ileocecal Valve (Figure 10.2) is the lower portion of the ileum at the junction of the cecum and the colon. A sphincter valve controls passage of the contents from the small intestine to the large intestine.

When the food reaches the large intestine, the digestible parts have already been acted on by enzymes, so basically the functions of the large intestine are absorption of water and elimination of mucus and waste products.

The large intestine can be divided into the ascending, transverse, descending and sigmoid areas of the colon. (**See Figure 10.3**)

The cecum—the first portion of the large intestine. The appendix is also located on the blind end of the cecum.

The colon—rises from the cecum as the **ascending** colon on the right side of the body; turns to become the **transverse** colon and then turns downward on the left as the **descending** colon. It then makes an "S" turn, forming the portion known as the **sigmoid flexure** part of the sigmoid colon. This is one of the Reflexologist's most difficult reflex areas to work. It then passes into the pelvic region to the level of the sacral vertebrae where it becomes the **rectum**.

ACCESSORY ORGANS TO DIGESTION

The main salivary glands are located just outside the mouth cavity. The saliva produced by these glands is about 98%

water, the balance being made up of inorganic salts and enzymes.

The one important enzyme is ptyalin which begins to digest the starches within the food by breaking them down into more simple forms of carbohydrate sugars.

THE LIVER

The liver is a secreting, spongy type organ weighing about three pounds; it has the ability to double its normal size under certain conditions. It is located predominately on the right side of the body in the upper area of the abdominal cavity below the diaphragm and protected by the rib cage. The liver performs over 500 functions and even takes over some of the functions of the spleen should the occasion arise. It also has the ability to regenerate itself in many cases. But most importantly: if the liver fails, the body dies.

Of chief importance is the liver's metabolic functions, including carbohydrate metabolism. This simply means the formation and storage of glycogen which the liver turns into glucose (a sugar) when it is needed and then releases it into the blood stream. The level of sugar into the blood is delicately balanced by one of the functions of the pancreas ... the release of the hormones insulin and glucagon. Insulin helps to prevent an abnormally high blood-sugar. If the pancreas does not secrete an adequate amount of insulin, the percentage of sugar in the blood causes the kidneys to react and they excrete excess sugar in the urine. As a result, the glycogen stored in the liver becomes depleted causing serious damage. Glucagon has an opposite function to that of insulin as it elevates blood-sugar when needed by accelerating the change of glycogen to glucose. (For a fuller discussion on diabetes, **See Chapter 12**, the Endocrine System.)

Cholesterol is an essential element of the blood, the precursor of hormones and is controlled in the blood stream by the thyroid. It is manufactured within the liver and is also absorbed from certain foods, including animal fats, egg yolk, butter, cream and milk, but it is not found in fruit, vegetables, cereals and nuts.

Today, there is evidence that emotional tension, in addition to its direct effect on the blood vessels, hastens the process of narrowing the coronary blood vessels by interfering with the metabolism of fats and overloading the blood stream with the fatty substance—cholesterol—which thickens the arteries.

Disturbances within the liver can be indicated by such conditions as continuing fatigue, irritability, sleeplessness and liver pains. To summarize this important organ's contribution to bodily health:

The liver aids in:

Digestion	Coagulation
Metabolism	Bile formation
Circulation	Detoxification
Blood formation	

It destroys poisons and microbes, detoxifies unwanted chemicals, and stores vital vitamins, glycogen, fats, carbohydrates, proteins and minerals, including iron and copper.

Special liver cells (Kupffer) clean intestinal blood before its re-entry into the general circulation. Dead body cells are changed into usable items such as bile. Small wonder that the liver reflex lists high in importance.

THE GALL BLADDER

The gall bladder is a muscular, pear-shaped receptacle for bile that is manufactured in the liver. It is attached to the underside of the liver and linked to the duodenum by a duct system. The duodenum is the first looping section of the small intestine.

Bile is secreted by the liver at about 500cc a day. It passes from the liver into a common bile duct. It sometimes enters the duodenum or into the gall bladder where it is stored.

Bile has, as one of its more important functions, the emulsification of fats, thus assuring their digestion and absorption. Another function of importance is that it serves as a lubricant in the intestines.

The walls of the gall bladder contain smooth muscles and in its hollow interior is stored some of the bile formed by the liver between meals. The entrance into the intestine of the gastric contents of the stomach (containing hydrochloric acid and fats) not only stimulates bile production by the liver but also causes previously formed bile to be expelled from the gall bladder into the duodenum.

THE PANCREAS

The pancreas functions as both an exocrine gland and an endocrine gland. As an exocrine gland, it aids in the digestion process. The digestive juice of the pancreas contains enzymes that break down proteins into amino acids, starch into sugar, and fat into a more soluble state. Pancreatic juice also alkalinizes to combat the acidity from the stomach.

Located below the liver and the stomach, the pancreas is about 6 inches (152.4mm) in length and weighs about 3 ounces (85.0 grams). It supplies the fuel to stoke cellular fires for everything from the batting of an eyelid, to the involuntary pumping stroke of the heart.

143

As an endocrine gland, the pancreas is responsible for the secretion of insulin and glucagon into the blood stream. The release of these hormones is related to the level of glucose (blood-sugar) in the body at any given time. The combined action of insulin and glucagon keeps the blood-sugar at the proper levels and assures that glucose is burned and supplied as needed.

WORKING THE DIGESTIVE SYSTEM
(*See Figure 10.4*)

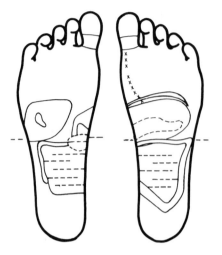

Figure 10.4

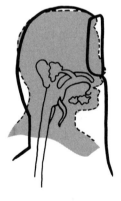

Figure 10.5

144

As we have previously indicated, digestion starts with the mouth or oral cavity.

Included with the mouth reflex will be the salivary glands which are arranged in pairs: the parotids (in the cheeks in front of the ears), the submandibulars (under the jaws) and the sublingual glands (under the tongue). To work these reflexes, look closely at *Figure 10.5*, where the face is superimposed on the great toes. The mouth reflex is usually found three quarters of the way from the tip of the toe downward. Slightly above and below this area will be the salivary glands reflexes. The throat reflex is located from the base of the toe upwards to where the fleshy or *ball* part of the toe starts. To effectively reach this reflex area, we have to work all the way around the toe. The bottom of the toe, of course, is the meaty part; the top of the toe is thinner and, therefore, is a very delicate area. Reflexologists will work all the way around the great toe as well as the sides of the toe. We, of course, work this area using both our thumb and finger techniques.

To start, the right thumb is used for the right foot; the left thumb for the left foot. Supporting the great toe, as shown in *Figure 10.6*, the thumb technique is used always with the forward motion. The fingers of the supporting hand are held around the great toe, as shown. Then, using the index

finger, we walk around the great toe
. . . and always with that forward
motion (**See Figure 10.7**). We also
work the same areas by coming **up**
and **down** the toes using both hands
in working the same toe.

We must remember that while working this reflex area on the great toe,
we are also working a multitude of
other reflexes. This region actually
represents the entire throat reflex
and, as I stated before, this area
includes a myriad of reflexes including the salivary glands, the
tongue, teeth and the esophagus, as
well as the tonsils and the thyroid
and parathyroids. Remember, the
small toes can be used for *fine-
tuning* this reflex. (I generally do not
work just this area—I usually work
from the base of the toenail to the
base of the great toe.)

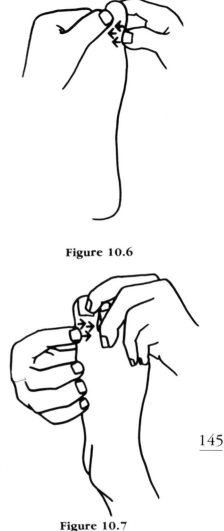

Figure 10.6

Note that when working this area, it
is not an *X marks the spot* type of
working. Also, we must remember
just how important it is to work the
entire region and not just one-half
of the throat, so we must work all the

Figure 10.7

145

way around the great toe of each foot searching for tender
reflex points.

ESOPHAGUS

Now, following our food, once it leaves the throat and is
swallowed, it is sent down the esophagus to the stomach.
Anatomically, our esophagus runs left of the midline. This
reflex will be found on the left foot. (**See Figure 10.8**) To
work this area, tip the foot out and begin with the right
thumb and start at the inside edge of the base of the great

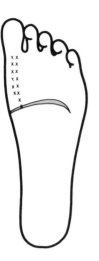

Figure 10.8

toe and work down toward the diaphragm line just outside the spine reflex. When reaching the diaphragm line, work with left thumb towards outside to a point where the diaphragm intersects the groove between the first and second toe (relative to the thyroid reflex). Where these two meet will be the reflex point for hiatus hernia, a protrusion of the upper stomach through the diaphragm. As a helper area, we would work the entire diaphragm reflex area on both feet for relaxation.

STOMACH

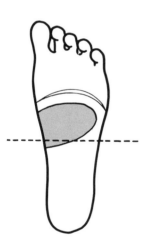

Figure 10.9

The largest part of the stomach reflex is going to be found on the left foot (**See Figure 10.9**). The stomach, of course, will also extend to the right foot because of its anatomical location within the body. Note that the stomach reflex itself is located below the diaphragm guideline of the foot and above the waist guideline.

As I previously mentioned, a part of the stomach's function is to change the chemistry of the swallowed food. So we should always thoroughly work the stomach reflex. Generally, we are going to start with our left hand on the left foot and work from the waistline in a criss-cross motion up to the diaphragm. The holding hand should be on the bottom of the foot with the fingers gently holding the toes. We must be careful here that we do not hold the great toe back when the area of the protruding tendon is being worked. Briefly release the pressure and then resume the original grip on the toe once the tendon area is passed over. Starting with

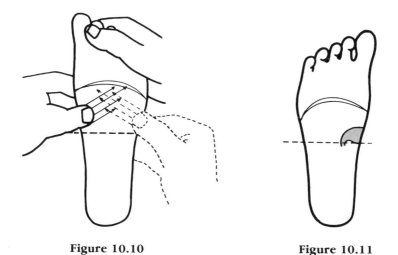

| Figure 10.10 | Figure 10.11 |

our left hand, using the thumb technique, we will cover the entire region. Then we will change hands and come back in the opposite direction, giving us the "criss-cross" effect. (*See Figure 10.10*).

Another important reflex is the duodenal area on the right foot. (*See Figure 10.11*.) We start with our right thumb and cover the reflex area above the waistline and half way to the diaphragm located from the first zone to about the third zone.

147

LIVER

Sequentially, the next area we will be working is the liver. The liver reflex, of course, will be on the right foot since the liver is located predominately in the right quadrant of our body. (*See Figure 10.12*.) The reflex area covers the space from the waistline to the diaphragm from the inside to the outside of the right foot. Being such, the reflex area will be extremely large; when working this area, we have to work it systematically and evenly. We start with our right hand and work the area towards the

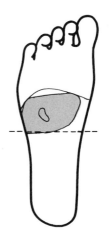

Figure 10.12

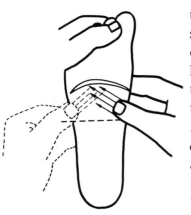

Figure 10.13

diaphragm with the holding hand on the toes and taking those nice and slow creeping motions. Then we come back over the area, change hands, and come across the area in the opposite direction angling towards the diaphragm (**_See Figure 10.13_**). _Remember to watch the tendon when crossing it, as described in the stomach reflex._ It is important as in any other reflex area, that when we are working the liver for any condition, we must make sure to work the **entire** area.

GALL BLADDER

Simultaneously, while working the liver reflex, we are going to be working the gall bladder reflex. The gall bladder is embedded within the liver, so naturally it is much smaller and the reflex area for it is sometimes varied.

Generally, the gall bladder reflex will be around the third or fourth zone above the waistline approximately half-way to the diaphragm (**_See Figure 10.12_**). This is not an easy reflex to find; sometimes when faced with someone afflicted with gall stones, you must systematically search for the reflex by coming in at different angles.

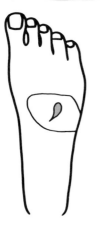

Figure 10.14

Occasionally, on a thin foot the gall bladder reflex can be located on the top of the foot just opposite the reflex site on the bottom of the foot. In other words, if you were to find the reflex on the bottom of the foot and then draw a line straight through the foot and come out on the top side, this area could also be worked. (**_See Figure 10.14_**)

Many times a person with gall bladder troubles can be worked much more effectively by working the reflex area on the top of the foot. This, of course, will be an extremely sensitive area. So it is important to note that, many times, when working the gall bladder and you have a problem locating the reflex, you should check the top of the foot. For some reason, the top of the foot is better on some people. But be aware that this is a bony area and extremely sensitive and a good reflex technique is necessary. (**See Figure 10.15**).

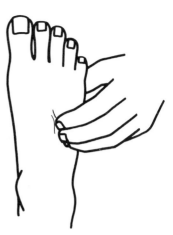

Figure 10.15

PANCREAS

The pancreas is located in the abdomen, behind the stomach and in front of the spine (**See Figure 10.16**). It is one of the busiest and most important glands in our body. This reflex area is one which must rank high in importance, so knowing how to work it efficiently and effectively is a must.

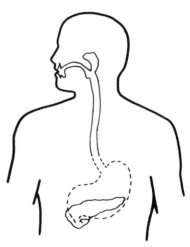

Figure 10.16

149

The reflex area for the pancreas is found on both feet, but mainly on the left. On the left foot, it is located slightly above the guideline to the waist to approximately half way to the diaphragm (**See Figure 10.17**). To work the area, we use our thumb technique in tiny caterpillar bites, being sure to hold the toes back with the holding hand as we work across this reflex. When reaching the protruding tendon, relax your hold on the toes, allowing the tendon to ease back into

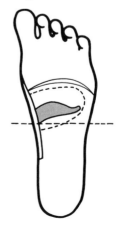

Figure 10.17

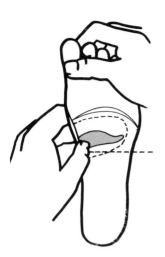

Figure 10.18

the foot for a moment until you pass over it. Push back and then continue to work across the entire region (**See Figure 10.18**). After several slow and complete passes from the initial direction, change hands and work in the same manner from the other direction. On the right foot the reflex will be slightly below the waist guideline.

REMEMBER: Just because the pancreas is located deep within the body, it does not mean that you have to dig deep within the foot to locate this reflex. In most cases, this area will be tender, so ease up on the pressure if this is the case. Remember there are overlapping organs in this region.

INTESTINES

Since the intestines occupy such a large area on both sides of the body, we will, or course, work both feet.

ILEOCECAL VALVE

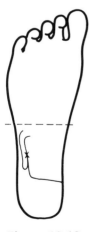

Figure 10.19

As you study **Figure 10.19**, note the area where the small intestine empties into the large colon . . . this area is an extremely important one to the Reflexologist since it is the location of the ileocecal valve. This is also an important reflex for the appendix (the appendix is in the area of the ileocecal valve).

NOTE: Tenderness in this area may indicate scar tissue, such as

an appendectomy scar . . . it does not always indicate problems.

As you develop your Reflexology skills, you will quickly note that scars and/or adhesions from previous surgery usually will show tenderness in their related anatomical areas. The ileocecal valve reflex is always worked by using the hook-in, back-up motion. (**See Chapter 4**). This reflex area is found on the bottom-outside (little toe side) of the right foot, below the waistline. To locate this reflex, I use the basic holding technique with the right hand and use my left thumb as the working hand, then run it down the outside edge of the right foot from the fifth metatarsal into the deepest part of the curve. When I locate this area, I take the thumb, bend it at the first joint and then use the hook-in, back-up technique. This reflex will be fairly close to the outside edge of the foot on the bottom between the fourth and fifth zone. (**See Figure 10.20**).

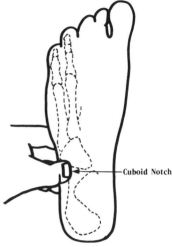

Figure 10.20

151

Once again, the fingers play an important part in giving us leverage by resting them on top of the foot. This maneuver gives the thumb the leverage it needs to work this difficult reflex area. Wrapping the fingers of the working hand around the foot, we hook-in and back-up.

SMALL AND LARGE INTESTINES

We will start on the right foot with the left holding hand on the bottom of the foot and the fingers gently wrapped over the toes, while pushing the great toe back with the thumb. We will be working the area from the waistline to the heel line of both feet for both the large and small intestines. Work across this area first with the right hand and then the left hand with our basic thumb technique in the criss-cross method. Now that we have worked this area over thoroughly, we will work in a pattern for the large colon.

Anatomically, as we look at the location of the large intestine, it outlines the small intestine. It comes up from the ileocecal valve reflex toward the little toe on the right foot. This area is referred to as *the ascending colon*:

(It should be noted that because the small intestine and the large intestine are so inextricably positioned that when working the reflex of the area, you are working both the large and small intestines.)

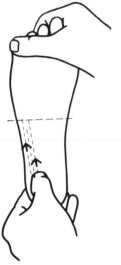

ASCENDING COLON

Working the ascending colon on the right foot, we use our left hand and "walk" in a forward motion toward the top of the foot, from the heel towards the waistline guideline, between the fourth and fifth zone. (***See Figure 10.21***). Repeat this process several times working in widening areas as shown.

Figure 10.21

TRANSVERSE COLON

The transverse colon sweeps across the abdominal cavity from right to left, below the stomach. When it reaches the spleen, it bends downward to become the descending colon. To work the transverse colon reflex, we will work across the waistline on both the right and left foot. The descending colon extends downward along the left side of the abdomen to the brim of the pelvis. From this point on, the colon courses in a curve like the letter "S" . . . called the sigmoid colon, or sigmoid flexure.

SIGMOID COLON

The way to locate the sigmoid flexure is to begin on the inside of the left foot where the heel guideline and the spine reflex intersect. Note: this area is also called the *bladder reflex*. From this point, we angle down at approximately 45 degrees to where the 3½ zone line intersects that angle. (**See Figure 10.22**).

It is imperative that before you try to make contact with this reflex, you should work the heel in several directions with both thumbs to soften up the area.

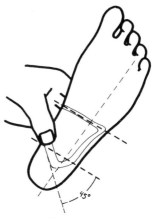

Figure 10.22

Tipping the foot out with your right holding hand, your left thumb will walk down the 45 degree angle from the heel line to where the lines intersect (3½ zone line) using the hook-in, back-up technique at the *cross hairs*. Your holding hand will be on the bottom of the foot with the fingers wrapped around the toes.

After using the left thumb for the hook-in, back-up technique and after working the whole line downward, you will change hands and use the right hand on the left foot, placing the heel of the left foot in the palm of the left hand.

Tip the foot out in a comfortable position and put the fingers of the working hand around the foot for leverage. (**See Figure 10.23**).

Starting at the heel line on the inside point, you work down at a 45 degree angle to this pinpoint reflex, stop, hook-in, back-up and then repeat the process several times, remembering always to come in at this angle.

153

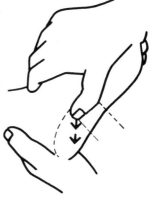

Figure 10.23

The reason for this specific angle is that experience has taught us that this specific angle is the **only** effective approach to a most difficult reflex. I have found that many people will ignore working this area because it is callused, thick, difficult to work, and very tiring. This is an important reflex and should be given the same attention as the other reflexes.

Diverticulitis and Colitis are some of the problems associated with the colon. The sigmoid flexure reflex is important for problems associated with gas. Often people with chest pains think they are having a heart attack, and find it to be a *gas pocket* initiated in the sigmoid flexure, backing up to the splenic flexure and thus pushing against the diaphragm. This causes pressure against the stomach and heart with subsequent discomfort in the heart area.

I have found that people with varicose veins often have colon problems and working the entire colon reflex may help this condition.

Constipation often starts in the sigmoid region because of a lack of exercise, low fiber diet or other contributing factors. When we think of colon problems or constipation, it is necessary that we do not just think of working the intestinal tract. Here is where our *helper areas* are important. Our key helper areas for constipation would be the liver because it produces and manufactures the bile, also the diaphragm— solar plexus because emotions have a great effect on our digestive system. But we must also think of working the adrenal glands, because the adrenals help us with muscle tone which in turn helps with the peristaltic action in the intestinal tract. Another area to think about is the lower back reflex for the nerves that supply the colon. These are the helper areas that are important to work along with the colon.

DESCENDING COLON

Once you have worked the sigmoid colon area several times, put your right hand and fingers beneath the heel, with the foot straight up, and the left holding hand on the metatarsals with the fingers over the toes. Place your right thumb on the sigmoid flexure reflex and work in a forward motion toward the little toes on the outer edge up to the waistline . . . this represents the descending colon. (**See Figure 10.24**).

It is important to note here that the primary reason that we go **up** the descending colon is because of the leverage advantage using the right hand. Many people say that we should *massage* the way the material in the colon flows.

Let me repeat, **Reflexology is not massage** . . . it makes no difference what direction you work . . . make several passes up between the regions of the 4th and 5th zones. It should be noted that anytime you are working the area from the waistline to the heel line, you are working the intestinal reflexes. And you must remember to come in at **all** angles. The two exceptions are the sigmoid flexure and the ileocecal valve . . . the sigmoid on the left foot and the ileocecal on the right . . . these two are specific pinpoint reflexes which use the hook-in, back-up technique.

RECTUM

The sigmoid reflex is very helpful for rectal problems caused by constipation. Constipation causes pressure and can result in hemorrhoids. While you are softening up the heel area in preparation to work the sigmoid flexure, you will be covering the rectal reflex. We also find that the lower back reflex is the helper area for rectal problems: the sacral-coccyx area particularly. Often, an injury to this area

155

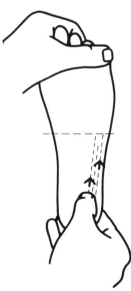

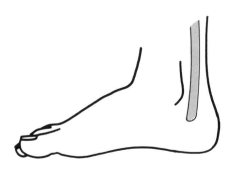

Figure 10.24   **Figure 10.25**

can affect the rectum. Another area I find helpful is working on the inside of the leg halfway between the Achilles tendon and the ankle bone in the hollow starting four to six inches above the ankle bone. We should gently walk the thumb down the groove on the leg formed between the Achilles tendon and the ankle bone. This reflex is called chronic prostate/uterus/rectum/sciatic. There are many reflexes located in this area (**See Figure 10.25**). Generally, lack of exercise adds to this problem. For working this reflex, refer to the Reproductive System.

To sum up: This chapter is an important one for any practicing Reflexologist: Refer to it often and practice its message repeatedly.

DISORDERS OF THE DIGESTIVE SYSTEM

DISORDER	DESCRIPTION	REFLEX AREAS TO WORK
Appendicitis	Inflammation of the vermiform appendix.	Ileocecal, diaphragm.
Cholesterol	A sterol widely distributed in animal tissues and occuring in the yolk of eggs, various fats and nerve tissues. It can be synthesized in the liver and is a normal constituent of bile. It is the principal constituent of most gall stones.	Thyroid, liver.
Cirrhosis	A chronic disease of the liver resulting in the loss of functioning liver cells and increased resistance of flow of blood through the liver.	Liver, pancreas, all glands.
Colitis	An inflammation of the colon.	Colon, liver, adrenals, lower spine, diaphragm, gall bladder.
Constipation	Difficult defecation.	Liver, gall bladder, diaphragm, adrenals, lower spine, sigmoid, ileocecal.
Diabetes	A disorder of the carbohydrate metabolism characterized by hyper-glycemia and glycosuria and resulting from inadequate production or utilization of insulin.	Pancreas, liver, all glands
Diarrhea	Frequent passage of watery bowel movements. A frequent symptom of gastrointestinal disturbances.	Ascending colon, transverse colon, diaphragm, liver, adrenals.
Diverticulitis	Inflammation of a diverticulum (little distended sacs) in the intestinal tract, especially in the colon which causes stagnation of the feces.	Colon, diaphragm, adrenals, lower spine, liver, gall bladder
Flatulence	Excessive gas in the stomach and intestines.	Intestines, stomach, liver, gall bladder, pancreas.

DISORDERS OF THE DIGESTIVE SYSTEM

DISORDER	DESCRIPTION	REFLEX AREAS TO WORK
Gall Stones	Stones formed in the gall bladder or bile ducts.	Liver, gall bladder, thyroid.
Hemorrhoids	A mass of dilated, tortuous veins in anus and rectum.	Diaphragm, adrenals, rectum, sigmoid, lower spine; also chronic area up back of heel.
Hernia	The protrusion or projection of an organ or part of an organ through the wall of the cavity which normally contains it.	Groin area, colon, adrenals.
Hiateal or Hiatus Hernia	Protrusion of the stomach upward into the cavity through the esophageal hiatus of the diaphragm.	Diaphragm, stomach, adrenal.
Hiccough	Spasmodic periodic closing of the glottis following spasmodic lowering of the diaphragm causing a short, sharp inspiratory cough.	Diaphragm, stomach.
Hypoglycemia	Deficiency of sugar in the blood.	Pancreas, liver, all glands.
Indigestion	Failure of the digestive function. Symptoms include heartburn, nausea, flatulence and cramps.	Liver, gall bladder, stomach, intestines, diaphragm.
Jaundice	A condition characterized by yellowness of skin due to deposition of bile pigments. It may be caused by obstruction of bile passageways, excess destruction of red blood cells, or disturbances in functioning of liver cells.	Liver
Phlebitis	Inflammation of a vein.	Adrenals, colon, liver; referral area: arm
Toothache	Self Descriptive.	All toes, middle 1/3 of great toes.

Tonsillitis	Inflammation of the tonsils.	Great toes, lymph system, all toes, adrenals, cervicals.
Ulcer	An open sore or lesion of the mucous membrane. A duodenal ulcer is located on the mucosa or lining of the duodenum due to the action of gastric juice. A peptic ulcer is located on the mucosa of the stomach.	Diaphragm, stomach, duodenum, reflex pertaining to location of ulcer.
Varicose Veins	Enlarged, twisted veins which may occur in almost any part of the body, but usually in the legs.	Colon, liver, adrenals; referral area: arm.

For a detailed listing of all disorders, see the charts at the back of this book.

Chapter 11

THE URINARY SYSTEM

"...They shall lay hands on the sick, and they shall recover."

Mark 16:18

THE URINARY SYSTEM

Your body has a waste collection system which would rival any in the world. A system that works around the clock to get rid of accumulated waste and toxins and to keep the internal environment within the body in a state of equilibrium.

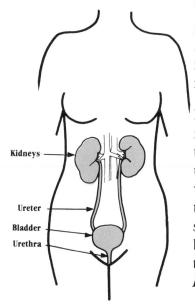

Kidneys

Ureter

Bladder

Urethra

Figure 11.1

The urinary system, of course, doesn't do it all. It has help in these functions through the lungs, skin and intestines ... they also play an important part in waste excretion.

But it is the urinary system which is responsible for the elimination of urine that carries most waste products from the cells, waste products which are carried to the kidneys in the blood stream. This intricate system consists of the kidneys, the bladder and the drainage tubes ... the ureters and the urethra. (***See Figure 11.1***).

The functions of the urinary system include:

- Maintenance of proper water balance in the body

- Ridding the body of toxic substances and other waste products, including nitrogen

- Keeping a proper concentration of salts and other substances in the blood

- Keeping a balance between acid and base in the body fluids

It should become increasingly clear that this system is extremely important to the Reflexologist. I constantly stress this to my seminar students and admonish them to always remember that this is the system which eliminates the toxins which are in the blood stream. If we are to maintain a proper balance within the body's systems, we are going to have to become very familiar with the urinary system and always remember to consider the importance of working these associated reflex areas.

The kidneys are the *master filters* of the body. It has been estimated that about one and one half quarts (1500 cc) of urine are usually excreted by the average adult every day. This filtering system is another of those remarkable aspects of the human body . . . the efficiency of the kidney filtering system can be demonstrated by the fact that it has a filtering capacity of a quart of blood per minute . . . 15 gallons an hour, or 360 gallons (1362.5 liters) a day. It usually filters from the blood about 180 quarts (170 liters) of fluid daily, returning usually 98% to 99% of the water, according to the needs of body.

The urine which is manufactured by the kidney filters contain, besides water, quantities of urea, uric acid, yellow pigments, amino acids and some minerals. The kidneys are important to remember when discussing gout, kidney stones, edema and high blood pressure.

As the urine is secreted, it leaves the kidneys and enters into the ureter tubes and then into the bladder. From the bladder, the urine is passed to the exterior of the body by the urethra.

Bladder infections are fairly common and usually more prominent in the female since the female urethra is shorter than the male and thus allows infectious organisms easier entry into the bladder. An inflammation of the bladder is called cystitis and is usually caused by bacteria. The kidneys, ureters, or bladder may form stones and this leads to painful and difficult urination.

As a Reflexologist, you will often encounter those persons who are suffering from kidney stones. These stones (called renal calculi) are usually composed of calcium oxalate, calcium carbonate, calcium, phosphate, or uric acid salts. Sometimes a stone made in the kidney will pass into the ureter tube causing intense pain (renal colic).

We can often help these people by careful attention to working the entire urinary system . . . bladder, ureters and, most importantly, the kidneys.

WORKING THE URINARY SYSTEM

I have noted that many Reflexologists work this system improperly or too hastily; there is a tendency to neglect concentration and needed effort on this reflex area. In my many conversations with seminar students, I find that one reason this system does not get its share of attention is that there are so many other organs and systems located within the same region. The students feel that this area has been worked every time the other systems are worked. This may be true when we recall the *packed suitcase* analogy, but it is not true when the person has a definite urinary problem. In this case, a deliberate effort to work the reflexes of the urinary system will be needed.

I continually stress the fact that a good Reflexologist should always picture the reflexes of the urinary system as they are projected onto the feet (*See Figure 11.2*).

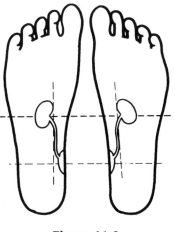

The urinary system reflexes will be located on both of the feet; the bladder being in the center of the body means that the bladder reflex will be found on the inside edge (medial) of both feet, above and below the heel guideline.

Figure 11.2

The kidney reflex is found in the center of the foot above and below the waistline guideline and on the outside of the tendon.

The ureters connect the kidneys to the bladder and are located on the inside of the tendon between the tendon and the spine reflex.

To work the urinary system, I will hold the right foot with the heel of the left hand on the metatarsal padding of the foot with the fingers over the small toes and with my thumb pushing against the great toe while tipping the foot in a comfortable outward position.

This technique will help to extend the tendon, a very important guideline for the ureter tubes.

I will use my basic thumb technique on the right foot. Using my right thumb, I will start at the bladder reflex and work across and up this reflex several times. With the same thumb, I will work through the bladder reflex over to the inside edge of the tendon and up the ureter tube reflex to the waistline alongside the tendon (**See Figure 11.3**). You can also work down this reflex with the left thumb. Then we will work in a forward motion either upward or across the kidney reflex on the outside of the tendon. It is extremely helpful to work both directions. In the case of kidney stones, I always recommend a high concentration of work on the ureter tube reflexes since this is where the stones usually get lodged. Most pain and consequent problems originate in these tubes.

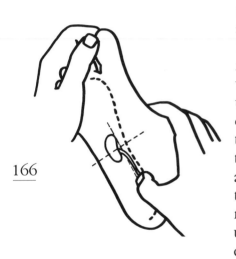

Figure 11.3

As for bladder infection, the Reflexologist's trained eye can usually spot chronic bladder problems because in many cases the reflex area will be a bit reddish and *puffy*. We always make sure to work this reflex as any infection of the kidneys can affect the bladder, and vice versa. A bladder infection can easily *back up* the tubes to the kidneys.

This process of working the urinary system on the right foot is then reversed when working on the left foot. I recommend that you work with your left hand for the reflex areas of the bladder, ureter tubes and the kidneys;

you could also use the right hand to work horizontally across the kidney reflex and down the ureter tube.

HELPER AREAS

The adrenal reflexes are helpful in cases of infection. For many of the back prolems associated with kidney malfunction, work the nerve reflexes coming off the spine. And remember that the parathyroids control calcium in the body and so it is a good helper area for kidney stones.

Another affliction, gout, was once called *the rich man's disease* for the simple reason that it was caused by rich foods and wine. It has also been called *metabolic arthritis* by the medical profession and for good reason since it is caused by too much uric acid which in turn results in a build-up of *urates* around the joints. Gout is marked by acute arthritis and an inflammation of one of the joints usually in the knee or foot. With gout, you should always thoroughly work the kidney reflexes.

Another affliction associated with the kidneys is one in which the kidneys themselves become inflamed. It is called either "Bright's disease," or Nephritis. This disease may afflict a portion of the kidney or the entire kidney itself, and may be acute or chronic. In any case, work the entire kidney reflex.

Another important problem associated with this system is called the *silent killer . . . hypertension* or high blood pressure associated with kidney disease. This disease is marked by a persistent elevation in the blood pressure and is due to a narrowing or blockage of the blood vessels. Some of the results of high blood pressure are cardiac hypertrophy and eventual heart failure; further hardening of the arteries; possible rupture of the blood vessels, especially those in the brain which cause cerebral hemorrhaging or *apoplexy*. Hypertension can also cause kidney failure or compromise the ability of the kidneys to remove toxic waste from the blood and maintain the fluid, electrolyte and acid-base relationship so necessary for homeostasis. To work the areas associated with high blood pressure, work the diaphragm/ solar plexus; as helper areas, work the kidneys and glands.

As I mentioned, this system is not one which should be just passed over. It is very important to the well being of the entire body and merits your full attention. Go back and study some of the more important aspects of this system; you will be glad you did.

DISORDERS OF THE URINARY SYSTEM

DISORDER	DESCRIPTION	REFLEX AREAS TO WORK
Anuria	Cessation of the production of urine by the kidneys.	Ureters, bladder, kidneys, adrenals, lower spine.
Cystitis	Inflammation of the bladder.	,,
Dysuria	Difficult or painful passage of urine.	,,
Incontinence	Inability to retain urine.	,,
Kidney Stones	Also called renal calculus. Small stones form in the kidney and pass through the ureter usually with intense pain called renal colic.	Ureters, kidneys, bladder, diaphragm, parathyroid.
Nephritis	(Also called Bright's Disease) an inflammation of the kidney.	Kidneys
Uremia	Toxic condition in which nitrogenous substances accumulate in the blood.	Kidneys, adrenals.

For a detailed listing of all disorders, see the charts at the back of this book.

Chapter 12

THE ENDOCRINE GLANDS

"Behold I will bring it health and healing."

Jeremiah 33:6

THE ENDOCRINE GLANDS . . .
the remote control organs

Many times during my Reflexology seminars, a sudden quizzical look comes over the faces in the audience when we begin to discuss the Endocrine System. Much has been written in the medical literature about these powerful little ductless glands which together constitute the Endocrine System. The *endocrine glands*, along with the *nervous system*, are responsible for most of the activities in the body.

I sometimes like to compare them to the thermostat in our homes . . . they are like those remote control devices which keep our houses at just the right temperature. These endocrine glands help the body to adapt to our environment; some of them are even essential to life itself as well as for the smooth operation of all the body's parts.

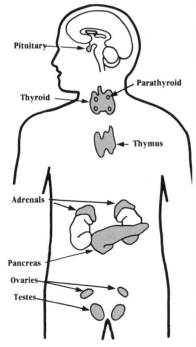

Figure 12.1

They are called *remote controls* for another simple reason: they are ductless and there are no direct "pipe lines" to one special organ. Rather, they produce internal secretions which are discharged into the blood stream or into the lymphatic system and then circulated to all parts of the body. The internal secretions produced by the endocrine glands are called **hormones** from the Greek *I stimulate*. Hormones produce profound effects on tissues and organs, many of them remotely located from the site of the origin of the hormone.

I always stress to my Reflexology students the importance of learning the anatomical location of these glands as shown in ***Figure 12.1***.

The endocrine glands are sometimes divided into three groups:

- The Pituitary (and the contiguous hypothalamus),

- The Thyroid, adrenals (suprarenals) and reproductive glands (ovaries and testes) which are under the control of the Pituitary,

- The parathyroid glands, pancreas, placenta and the gastrointestinal mucosa.

Now, let's take a closer look at these glands and their specific functions.

The main Endocrine Glands which you will be concerned with are:

- The Pituitary, or Master Gland

- The Parathyroid

- The Thyroid

- The Adrenals

- The Reproductive Glands

- The Pancreas

Other endocrine glands with which you should become familiar are ones whose contributions to bodily health are still relatively unknown. They include the thymus and the pineal body. The thymus is a two-lobed ductless gland located behind the upper part of the sternum. Large in children, it shrinks in size during adulthood. Sometimes considered an endocrine gland, it also has the structure of a lymph node and we discuss it further in the Lymphatic (*Chapter 7*). The thymus is important in the development of immune response during early childhood so that it helps to protect the young body from infectious disease. The Pineal body is located deep within the central part of the brain and is believed to be an endocrine gland whose specific function is still disputed today.

I must emphasize here that most of these glands are small, are located deep within the body, and usually lie within the first and second zones of the body.

THE PITUITARY

This gland is a rounded body about the size of a pea. It is attached to the hypothalamus at the base of the brain but it has a masterful part to play in the functioning of the body.

The Pituitary has been termed: the *master gland of the body, general headquarters* of the Endocrine system, and even *the leader of the endocrine orchestra*. It is easy to understand the reasoning behind all of these titles when you realize that this tiny gland is the only one which produces a hormone that specifically affects all of the other glands. As a matter of fact, it actually monitors the activities of the other glands.

Its basic hormones control skeletal growth, growth and development of the gonads, maturation of the reproductive cells and secretion of milk by the mammary glands. It also controls the functional activity of the thyroid, the islets of Langerhans in the pancreas, the adrenal cortex and often the parathyroids. This gland also plays an important function in controlling blood pressure.

I have found the Pituitary reflex excellent for reducing fevers and also useful in fainting spells. This gland is also responsible for cellular growth and it should be worked in all cases of extracellular growth whether the growth be benign or malignant.

The pituitary is also responsible for body growth . . . how tall or short you are. It should be worked as a normal procedure in all children.

THE PARATHYROIDS

These little glands, usually four in number, lie within the capsule of the thyroid gland and they are chiefly concerned with the metabolism of calcium and phosphorous and they

174

thereby keep the skeletal system in order. They also affect the nervous and muscular tissues.

They are very essential to life itself and sometimes a malfunction of the parathyroids causes the calcium and phosphorous of the bones to be carried away in the blood stream with the consequent effect that the bones become light, porous and brittle. This is a helper area for nerves and muscles of the body and also for kidney stones.

THE THYROID

The thyroid straddles the windpipe in the midportion of the neck. Each of the two lobes of this gland are connected by a narrow isthmus. The functions of this gland are to regulate the basal metabolism (the speed at which our body burns and uses cells), influence the body's growth, help in the development of the teeth, enhance muscle tone, aid in mental development, and to promote the functional activity of the gonads and the adrenal glands. Practically all of the iodine found in the body is found in this gland and so this reflex is especially important to work since most of that iodine is in the form of an amino acid and is responsible for stimulating the oxidative processes in the tissues of the body. It is also important to work this reflex for weight loss, nervousness, rapid heart beat, overweight problems and dryness of the skin. It is also excellent for the control of the cholesterol level of the blood and for mental sluggishness. This gland has also been called *the third ovary* because of its important affect on those glands in the female.

175

THE ADRENALS

The adrenals are sometimes called *suprarenals* as both names indicate location: *above the kidneys.* They are a pair of flattened, yellowish organs about two inches high, one inch wide and about one-half inch thick and are located right above each kidney.

The blood stream is very kind to these two glands since the aorta pumps a rich supply to them, and no wonder when you learn of their importance in body functioning.

We always look at the adrenals with their structure as well as their function in mind, since each gland is composed of two organs . . . a convoluted cortex surrounding a medulla.

In embryological development, the adrenal cortex gives origin to the sex glands. The cortex secretes about 50 hormones concerned with bodily strength and sex development. These hormones are divided into three groups:

- The body's own internal cortisone-like compounds which regulate sugar metabolism and combat inflammation;

- Electrolyte-regulating hormones that control sodium and potassium and water balance; and

- Sex hormones that supplement those secreted by the gonads.

The medulla secretes the important hormone adrenalin (epinephrine), the activator which works on the nervous system.

Stressful situations such as worry, anger, or fear increase the flow of adrenalin which, in turn, prepares the body for *flight or fight* by initiating:

- An immediate rise in blood pressure;

- Stepped up respiration rate;

- Stimulation of the skeletal muscles thus increasing the capacity for work;

- Increase in the basal metabolism rate and the rate of oxygen consumption; and

- Increased blood sugar by stimulating the liver to release glucose from glycogen.

The adrenals are responsible for giving us what I am fond of calling the old *giddy-up-and-go*. When a person is run down and apathetic all the time . . . look to the adrenals.

Adrenalin also helps to give us the muscle tone we need throughout the body, including that important peristaltic action in the intestines. Adrenalin is also important in the treatment of heart problems as well as asthma.

The importance of adrenalin in checking attacks of asthma can be emphasized by anyone who has had a severe attack . . . the emergency procedure to restore normal breathing is a shot of adrenalin. Relief comes almost immediately.

THE GONADS OR REPRODUCTIVE GLANDS

The testes and the ovaries secrete into the blood stream certain substances which control the appearances of the secondary sex characteristics. (These are fully covered in the Reproductive Organs *Chapter 13*).

THE PANCREAS

I lightly covered the pancreas in the Digestive System (*Chapter 10*). But, it might be wise to reiterate here, that the pancreas is located behind the stomach. It lies in a horizontal position, the *head* attached to the duodenum, the *tail* reaching to the spleen. The larger portion is found above the waist guideline on the left foot and the smaller portion will be slightly below the waist guideline on the right foot.

And remember that the pancreas produces both external and internal secretions. The external secretion, called pancreatic juice, contains alkalinizing bicarbonate and digestive enzymes. The internal secretions are hormones called insulin and glucagon that come from masses of cells called *islets of Langerhans* scattered throughout the gland.

Insulin and glucagon play a primary role in the regulation of carbohydrate metabolism, including the use of glucose by the tissue cells as well as the formation and conversion of glycogen into glucose in the liver.

WORKING THE ENDOCRINE GLANDS

PITUITARY GLAND

I always recommend examining the great toe when you begin to work the pituitary reflex. Why? Well, Mother Nature has made toes in all shapes and sizes, and since the pituitary reflex represents one of the *target* areas in which we will be using the *pinpointing* technique, you must *know the toe*.

After years of experimenting, I have developed a special measuring technique which will enable you to pinpoint the pituitary reflex. To accomplish this, I always look for the widest point on both sides of the great toe and then I draw an imaginary line from point to point. Now, there will be many times when you will find that this wide point may be callused, and you will use this callused area for your measurement. Once you have the line drawn, the pituitary reflex will be found at the mid-point of this hypothetical line. As I have previously stated, the configuration of many great toes will be somewhat different; some lines will run straight across the toe while others may be slightly slanted. This mid-point should be close to the center of the great toe. (**See Figure 12.2**).

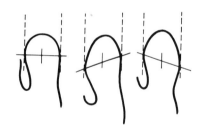

Figure 12.2

Now, to the actual working of this reflex area.

First, I determine just what hand/foot combination is best for this reflex. I have found that it is important when working the right foot that I use the right hand, and on the left foot I use the left hand. The holding hand will be used to protect and support the great toe. I always cover the toes with the fingers of the holding hand; I use the fingers of the working hand for leverage. The leverage fingers are always on the outside of the holding hand. This is done to prevent any injury or unnecessary pain to the top of the great toe.

To work the pituitary reflex area, we always use the inside corner of the thumb on the working hand by utilizing the *hook-in, back-up* technique . . . remember the *bumblebee* who sits down and backs up? (**See Figure 12.3**). Be sure to start this *hook-in, back-up* a little beyond the midpoint so that when you pull back you will be directly over the reflex point. I use this technique with a very slight rotation on the pin point reflex. (**See Technique Chapter 4**).

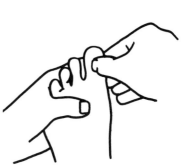

Figure 12.3

I generally recommend making three or four working contacts with this reflex area and coming back later to repeat this technique.

WORKING THE THYROID AND PARATHYROID

Since the thyroid gland is located at the base of the neck area, the reflex area will be located at the base of the great toe.

To work this area effectively, I always recommend holding and protecting the great toe with the holding hand. I use the

thumb of the holding hand to hold the toe so that it may be worked on effectively by the thumb of the working hand. And I always place the fingers of the working hand on those of the holding hand.

Using the basic thumb technique (as shown in **Figure 12.4**), I make several passes, walking across the base in one direction, change hands, and come back in the opposite direction in the same manner. This, of course, is done in order to completely cover the comparatively wide

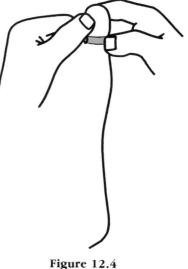

Figure 12.4

reflex area for the thyroid. Working several passes in one direction and then changing hands to work in the opposite direction will give you complete coverage of the thyroid reflex area. This will also include the parathyroids since they are buried in the thyroid.

HELPER AREA

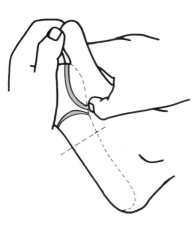

Figure 12.5

A helper area for the thyroid is working between the great toe and the second toe on the bottom of the foot. Start where the diaphragm and the spine intersect and work under the great toe joint and then up the groove between the great toe and second toe. (**See Figure 12.5**). Start with the right hand making several passes. This helps relax the upper back, throat and nerves in this area. We could also work the top of the foot between the great toe and the second toe.

WORKING THE ADRENAL GLANDS

As I previously mentioned, the adrenals are located on top of each kidney. I have already discussed the supreme importance of these glands . . . including the fact that they give us what I am fond of referring to as *the giddy-up-and-go*. Actually, the adrenals have over fifty functions to perform.

The reflex areas for the adrenals are somewhat complex. Although they lie atop the kidneys, they are in no way related to them. The adrenal reflexes can be located in the area halfway between the waistline and the diaphragm line, on the inside and next to the protruding tendon.

I always work the adrenal reflex area by holding the foot with the heel of the holding hand on the metatarsal padding and the thumb on the great toe, which, when pushed back, extends the tendon for a landmark.

I always recommend using the right hand to work on the right foot and the left hand for working on the left foot. Using the basic thumb technique, I walk slowly from the waist line toward the diaphragm line. When I am approximately half-way up this area, I usually find a very sensitive area (adrenal reflex) on the inside of the foot right next to the protruding tendon (**See Figure 12.6**). You can also tip the foot out and with your left thumb work down this same area. This area is often very tender, so be sure to ease up a bit on the pressure when you find this type of situation.

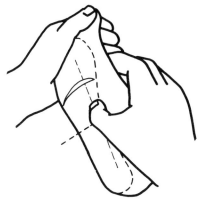

Figure 12.6

I sometimes use the reflex rotation technique as I work this all important reflex. I have developed this special *pivot* hold for this reflex, which I find works quite effectively. I hold the thumb on the exact reflex area and then flex the foot back and forth on the pivot of the thumb. (**See Technique Chapter 4**).

181

PANCREAS

The reflex area for the pancreas is found on both feet (**See Figure 12.7**) but mainly on the left one. On the left foot it is located from the guideline to the waist to about halfway to the diaphragm. To work this area, we use our basic thumb technique in tiny caterpillar bites, being sure to hold the toes back with the holding hand as we work across this reflex. When reaching the protruding tendon, relax your hold on the toes

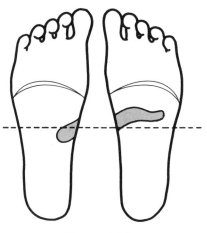

Figure 12.7

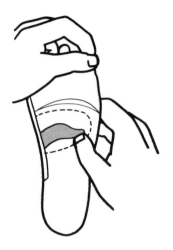

Figure 12.8

allowing the tendon to ease back into the foot for a moment until you pass over it. Then continue to work across the entire region several times (*See Figure 12.8*).

After several slow and complete passes from the initial direction, change hands and work in the same manner from the other direction (*See Figure 12.9*). On the right foot, the reflex will be slightly below the waist guideline. Work in the same manner as for the left foot.

One of the main concerns you will have when working the pancreatic reflex is, of course, diabetes. As a Reflexologist, the first question we ask of a diabetic is, "*How long have you had diabetes?*" There is a rationale in asking this since Reflexology has had its best results with those who have acquired diabetes later in life. This type of diabetes is generally believed to have been initially caused by trauma or shock of some kind. Diabetes is also covered in ***Chapter 10***.

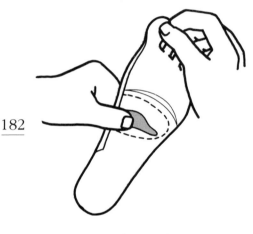

Figure 12.9

The pancreas is one of those organs very susceptible to shock and so, using Reflexology techniques, we have had favorable results with normalizing the pancreas simply by reducing that tension which initially caused the problem.

A diabetic who has suffered from childhood may have inherited it but allergy to self (auto immunity of the pancreas) is known to be involved. This type of condition is more difficult and must be worked on much longer.

A word of caution: Often when working this type of diabetes it is easy to become discouraged since we see no immediate results . . . sometimes it takes months before any results are evident. Generally, the Reflexologist can often help the diabetic with their circulatory and adjunctive problems. Keeping all of the benefits in mind, make sure that you apply a thorough working of both feet; this will help regardless of whether or not the insulin unit dosage comes down. Improving circulation is worth all of our efforts.

Another potential problem in working the diabetic: oftentimes they have lost feeling in the foot area. Even when there is no feeling you should work the pancreatic reflex as well as all the other reflexes.

In the case of the childhood diabetic, you must consider the fact that perhaps the pancreas stopped growing at an early age . . . when the person becomes a little older and more active, the body needs more insulin and the pancreas just cannot keep up with the demand. The Reflexologist cannot help the pancreas to produce the amount needed, but, since the child is still growing, we might be able to assist nature and get the pancreas normalized so that it can continue growth, however small. And, if they are on insulin, less insulin may be required. If insulin dosage can be reduced, however slightly, we are accomplishing something.

183

Do not at any time recommend that they alter their medication without first consulting their physician.

Diabetics are sometimes difficult to work with, often for a variety of reasons. Many times they will not stay on their diet if feeling better. Or, when their tests show a slight improvement, they may lower their medication dosage. Always encourage the diabetic to keep in contact with their physician and inform him of any planned change in either diet or medication.

Again, I cannot stress enough the importance of establishing a regular working schedule for the diabetic. I recommend working the diabetic on a regularly established schedule for two, three, or even four times a week. Working a short period of time each day would be best even if they were to do their own homework.

And a few words on the opposite of **hyper**glycemia: **hypo**glycemia. Hypoglycemia is described as an abnormally low blood glucose level and is usually caused by a rapid and excessive removal of glucose from the blood or from a decreased secretion of glucose into the blood. Overproduction of insulin usually causes this condition. For a complete and clear overview of the whole problem of blood sugar levels, I always recommend my students reading:

Sugar and Your Health
by Ray C. Wunderlich, Jr., M.D.
Johnny Reads, Inc. 1982
Box 12834
St. Petersburg, Florida 33733, U.S.A.

In cases of hypoglycemia, (low blood sugar) and hyperglycemia, be sure to work the pancreas and the liver.

The Endocrine glands are extremely important in regulating the body's delicate balance. Remember all the glands work together and help one another. Be sure you are familiar with them, their function, and their location.

Chapter 13

THE REPRODUCTIVE SYSTEM

"The fruit of the womb is his reward"

Psalms 127:3

THE REPRODUCTIVE SYSTEM

Life itself is sacred . . . a God given gift to every living thing on this green earth. And, consequently, every living thing has a means of reproducing itself in order to perpetuate the species.

With humans, the reproductive system in the male and the female consists of the primary sex organs, the testes and the ovaries which produce the sex cells called the spermatozoa and ova. The accessory sex organs have the primary function of uniting the sex cells and then the protection and nourishment of the developing embryo. Also important: the hormones which are produced by these glands and which ultimately influence bodily development and behavior.

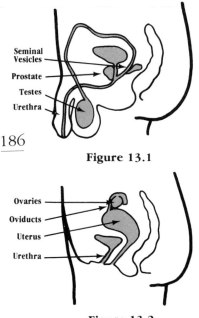

Seminal Vesicles
Prostate
Testes
Urethra

Figure 13.1

Ovaries
Oviducts
Uterus
Urethra

Figure 13.2

The male reproductive system consists of the testes, the duct system including the urethra (the duct which leads from the bladder to the outside of the body).

The male accessory reproductive glands include the seminal vesicles and the prostate gland. The prostate is that gland which surrounds the neck of the bladder and the urethra in the male. (**See Figure 13.1**).

In the female, the primary organs of reproduction are the ovaries. The accessory organs are the Fallopian tubes (or oviducts), the uterus and the mammary glands (the breasts). (**See Figure 13.2**).

Both testes and ovaries serve two functions:

- The production of reproductive cells.

- The production of hormones.

The hormones which stimulate the development of male characteristics are called androgens. The hormones which stimulate the development of female characteristics are called estrogens.

The most potent androgenic substance produced by the testes is the principal hormone testosterone which, among other things, affects growth of hair, enlargement of the larynx resulting in a deeper voice, development of height and form and the development of accessory glands, i.e., the prostate and seminal vessels.

The ovaries are the source of the estrogens which are essential for growth and form as well as to the normal functioning of the genital system. They also regulate cyclic changes in the uterus.

In children, we find these reflexes to be helpful in allergy cases and should always be worked. They have a lot to do with our well being and health before puberty and also after the reproductive years of life.

WORKING THE
REPRODUCTIVE SYSTEM

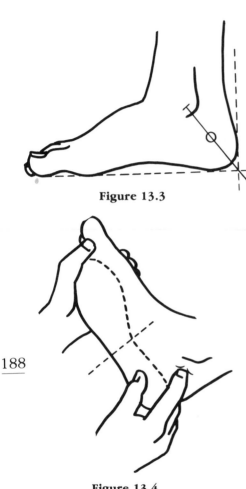

We will locate the uterus or prostate reflex on the inside (great toe side) half-way from the ankle bone to the back corner of the heel. To find this reflex, we take the high point of the ankle bone on the inside, square off the back edge of the heel, draw an imaginary line between these two points and then divide that line in half. This is where the uterus or the prostate reflex is found. (*See Figure 13.3*).

Figure 13.3

188

To work this reflex on the right foot, I make direct contact on this reflex area with my index finger of my right hand and use a slight circular motion (*See Figure 13.4*). We can also use our middle finger in this area.

Another method for working this reflex is to rest the right heel in the palm of the left hand, the middle finger on the left hand will be held gently on this reflex area. The thumb of the left hand will be wrapped around the outside part of the ankle where the ankle is joined onto the foot (groin area). Then place the heel of the right hand on the bottom of the foot at the metatarsal area and rotate the foot back and forth in a slight oval motion four or five times in one direction and then the same number of times in the opposite direction while con-

Figure 13.4

trolling the pressure with the middle finger (*See Figure 13.5*). ***This is a relaxing technique*** as well as a working one. This area is very sensitive and must be worked in a special way. Many times, you can easily miss this reflex point if you don't measure properly. This is one of the pin point areas and must be treated as such. Many ankles have a small indentation in this reflex area so look for it as a guideline. Repeat these procedures on the left foot with alternate hands.

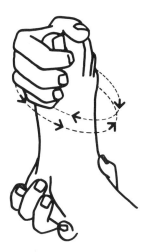

Figure 13.5

The ovary and the testicle reflex is found in the same manner as the uterus and prostate reflex except that it is found on the outside (little toe side). Find the high spot on the ankle bone, square off the back of the heel and draw an imaginary line; divide this line in half. This is where the ovary or testicle reflex is found. It is best to use your left index finger on the right foot. Place the finger on this spot where the lines cross and use that slight circular motion (*See Figure 13.6*). Repeat this on the left foot using the right hand. We do not

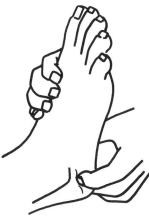

Figure 13.6

do the ankle rotation technique for this reflex as the contour of the hand and ankle is not conducive to this maneuver. Good helper areas for the ovaries are the thyroid, pituitary and adrenal reflexes.

To work the reflex area for the fallopian tubes in the female and the seminal ducts in the male, we will work where the foot is joined on to the leg at the ankle (where the foot bends). Remember, the fallopian tubes connect the ovaries to the uterus so visualize this on the foot. The uterus is on the inside of the ankle, the fallopian tube goes across the ankle from the inside to the outside where the ovaries are found.

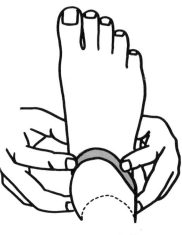

Figure 13.7

To work this reflex, we hold the foot up straight and work with the index fingers of both hands. Hold the heel of the foot on the Achilles tendon with the finger tips you are not using. Place both thumbs on the bottom of the foot in order to hold the foot up straight for control and support. Using both index fingers, walk up the groove formed where the foot joins the leg. Do not pinch the skin! When the fingers come close together, use only one finger at a time (**See Figure 13.7**). The thumbs can also be used one at a time. The client should be reminded to relax the foot and ankle. Never pull the foot forward to see what you are doing as this will tighten the area and not allow you to reach this reflex properly.

A nice relaxing technique for this area is called the **ANKLE ROTATION.** Place the webbing found between the thumb and the index finger of the left hand over the ankle of the right foot making sure that all fingers are kept together on the leg. The hand should fit the groove between the leg and the foot. **DO NOT SQUEEZE TOO HARD.** Using the right hand on the bottom of the foot, and holding the left hand firm, I rotate the foot four or five times in one direction, and then four or five times in the opposite direction (**See Figure 13.8**). This will help with swelling in the ankles as well. Remember: this area is also for the lymphatic system and anything in the groin area.

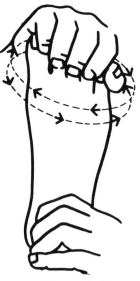

Figure 13.8

A most beneficial helper area for chronic prostate, uterus, rectum and sciatic problems is found in the area of the Achilles tendon. To work this area on the inside of the right foot, it is best to tip the foot out and push back with your left hand. Wrap the right hand around the lower part of the leg, about six inches above the ankle, and walk the

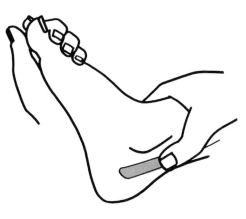

Figure 13.9

thumb down toward the heel in the Achilles tendon area at the inside back of the leg (**See Figure 13.9**). This area can be very sensitive so be sure to work it very gently and only to a tolerable threshold. There will be a natural groove formed by the tibia bone in this area, so I work this area all the way down to the uterus/prostate reflex. I find that working down is better than working up because we often have a tendency of pinching with our fingers on the outside of the leg.

This reflex area is excellent for prostate problems, menopause, menstrual problems, hemorrhoids, and sciatica.

191

The mammary glands (breasts) are also part of the reproductive system. When you are working this reflex area, you are also working the lung/chest area. The breast reflex is best worked on the top of the foot from the base of the toes to the diaphragm guideline. The working of this area is found under the Respiratory System **Chapter 9**. This reflex area is helpful for lumps and soreness in the breasts. Helper areas include the pituitary and the entire lymphatic system.

A WORD ABOUT PREGNANCY

Reflexology has been found to be quite helpful during the entire gestation period. In my opinion, and from my experience over the years, it will help for some of the associative problems of pregnancy including edema and morning sickness. It is also very helpful in relaxing the entire body during the actual delivery period. I have found it is beneficial to work on the person on a regularly scheduled basis during pregnancy.

And while on the subject of pregnancy, we have found that Reflexology has proved to be very beneficial as an aid in fertility. We have logged several scientific recordings of how sperm count has increased as a result of Reflexology!

Of course, this subject leads us to another about which we receive many questions during our seminars . . . the question of hysterectomies.

Hysterectomy is, of course, the removal of the uterus and is often accompanied by removal of the ovaries. There is often some surgical *shock* to the basal system. If a person is scheduled for this type of surgery, it is very advantageous to work **before** the scheduled surgery and also immediately after. An important thing to remember is that the estrogen supply is diminished when the ovaries are removed. The adrenal glands must compensate for this. It is important to work the adrenal reflexes as well as the thyroid and the pituitary in order to stimulate the needed hormones. The adrenals are ideal helper areas as is the thyroid gland and the pituitary gland. You will also note that all endocrine glands are very tender in a person who has had a hysterectomy.

Study the following chart for symptoms you can help with in this all important area.

DISORDERS OF THE REPRODUCTIVE SYSTEM

DISORDER	DESCRIPTION	REFLEX AREAS TO WORK
Hysterectomy	The operation for removal of the uterus and sometimes the ovaries and oviducts.	Adrenals, thyroid, pituitary, uterus, ovaries, fallopian tubes, diaphragm, chronic uterus area.
Impotence	Lack of power: chiefly of copulative power of virility.	Reproductive system, all glands, whole spine, diaphragm.
Infertility	Not able to conceive or induce conception.	Same as impotence.
Lump in Breast	Swelling of the lymphatic tissue in the breast.	Chest/lung, lymph system, pituitary.
Menopause (hot flashes)	When the body flushes during the change of life.	Diaphragm, all glands, reproductive system, chronic uterus area.
Menstrual Cramps	Self descriptive	Reproductive system, lower spine, all glands, diaphragm.
Morning Sickness	Feeling of nausea during pregnancy.	All glands, diaphragm, stomach
Ovaries (Cysts)	A foreign growth in the ovary.	Reproductive system, pituitary, all glands.

DISORDERS OF THE REPRODUCTIVE SYSTEM

DISORDER	DESCRIPTION	REFLEX AREAS TO WORK
Pre-natal care	Healthful care during pregnancy.	All glands, whole spine, diaphragm, bladder, reproductive system.
Prostate problems	Inflammation/enlargement of the prostate gland.	Reproductive glands, bladder, lower spine, pituitary, adrenals, chronic prostate area.

For a detailed listing of all disorders, see the charts at the back of this book.

Chapter 14

SUGGESTED PROCEDURE FOR A REFLEXOLOGY SESSION

"And that ye study to be quiet, and to do your own business, and to work with your own hands, as we command you;"

1 Thessalonians 4:11

SUGGESTED PROCEDURE FOR A REFLEXOLOGY SESSION

We have developed this book by discussing the various systems of the human body and the reflexes associated with those systems. This is done only to acquaint you with the human body and unless you are a physician this **should not** be discussed with your clients during a session. **We are not physicians nor do we take the place of a physician!** Because of the importance of this fact, let me add a few other admonitions:

We do not combine our work with the selling of other items . . . this could be construed as prescribing and we **never, in any instance, prescribe anything!**

Nor do we treat for specific conditions. Reflexology helps the body to establish homeostasis . . . to seek a natural balance between the systems. I would caution you to reread the above and to always let it serve as your professional guideline.

REMEMBER: If your client has a specific medical problem and has not seen his physician, you should recommend that he do so.

Before beginning make sure your nails are short and if your hands or their feet are perspiring, you may use corn starch (corn flour) or baby powder.

Now, let me suggest to you the most logical steps in working the feet during a Reflexology session.

If your client is new, remember to *meet the feet*. Always check for corns, calluses, ingrown toenails, or any other area which might cause discomfort through direct contact.

I always find it best to begin all sessions by initially using all the relaxing techniques on the feet to relax the client and to get their feet accustomed to my hands (***see Technique Chapter 4***). I also work the diaphragm-solar plexus reflex to further relax the client.

DIAPHRAGM TO BASE OF TOES

I will begin working with my right hand on the bottom of the right foot in the metatarsal area—the chest-lung reflex area.

After working this area thoroughly with both hands, I will work this same chest-lung area on the top of the foot with my index finger. Remember to work both the top and the bottom from the base of the toes to the diaphragm and from the inside of the foot to the outside. Be sure to work the shoulder reflex all around the little toe joint while you are in this area. Another important area, while you are in this section, is between the great toe and the second toe.

ALL TOES

Now that the client is accustomed to my hands, I proceed up to the toe reflex area. Starting with the great toe, I will work the cervicals, thyroid, side of the neck, brain, and pituitary making sure to work the whole great toe very carefully and systematically. Then on to the small toes covering the center and both sides from the tip to the base.

The toes are very sensitive so remember to start lightly and gradually increase the pressure.

197

EYE AND EAR

Next we will work the eye and ear reflexes at the base of the small toes. Remember to pull the padding down and "walk the ridge" with the outside edge of the thumb.

As you are working be sure to use your relaxation techniques often to keep the client more relaxed. If you don't, they will tense up.

DIAPHRAGM TO HEEL LINE

The next area to be worked is the soft tissue area of the foot between the diaphragm and the heel. This area contains most all the major organs so remember to work this area systematically from all angles. It is a must to have nice, smooth, even pressure or you will miss some important areas. Do not forget the special techniques for the ileocecal valve on the right foot.

HEEL AREA

Now we are down to the heel area where it is tough and callused. You will need good leverage and technique to work this area. This area is for the lower back, spurs in the heel, the rectum and also the sciatic nerve which passes under the heel. The sigmoid flexure (found on the left foot) is very important, so remember the 45° angle and the *hook-in, back-up* technique.

SPINE

As we have been working the sections down the foot we have also been working the spine reflex in each section.

As the spine is so important to the whole body, I like to work the whole spine reflex from the base of the heel to the top of the great toe. I will then change hands and work down this area. If there is tenderness in a specific area I will usually work across this area to be sure I have covered it thoroughly.

ANKLE AREA

Now I will work around the ankle for the reproductive system reflexes, the uterus-prostate on the inside, then the ovaries-testes on the outside and the fallopian tubes (this area is also for the groin and lymphatics). While we are in this area, on the outside of the ankle bone, I will work the hip-sciatic reflex under the ankle bone and the hip-knee-leg reflex in front of the ankle bone on the outside.

Last but not least is the chronic rectum-prostate-uterus-sciatic reflex on the inside of the leg. Be sure you work down the groove on the inside of the leg to the uterus-prostate reflex, (it is usually better working down the leg than up the leg).

A good Reflexologist will maintain contact at all times with the foot throughout this whole process.

After thoroughly working the one foot, change to the opposite one; work the second foot in the same sequence as described above.

When completed, return to the foot you first worked and concentrate on any tender spots you may have found. Then return to the second foot and work those tender spots.

I always recommend ending the session with relaxing techniques since this leaves the client with a wonderful relaxed feeling. My favorite one to finish a session with is the metatarsal kneading.

SOME HELPFUL HINTS

I have found that it is very beneficial when working a full session to always use a relaxing technique between each section of reflexes. For instance, after working the toes, I always use the side-to-side relaxer. You will find that this is very helpful, particularly on a sensitive foot. The more sensitive a person is, the more the relaxing techniques should be used. Just remember to use that relaxer which is appropriate to the region you are working. If you will go back and glance at the relaxing techniques we have discussed in *Chapter 4*, you will find that the choice for each reflex area is an easy one.

I am often asked why we work one whole foot and then change and work the entire other foot. We have found that when the entire foot is worked systematically, it actually feels better and allows you to really become acquainted with the anatomy of the foot upon which you are working. There is also a better pattern of performance and you will not miss any areas this way. To make it clear: you are actually *programming* your technique into a standard pattern that systematically covers every area of the foot.

Experience has shown that the client benefits more when it is done this way and it feels much better than constantly switching from one foot to the other.

THE LENGTH OF TIME FOR EACH SESSION?

The average session is usually 30 to 40 minutes and can, of course, vary with your experience as an operator. An initial session with a new client could take up to an hour since you will need to indoctrinate the person with the basics of Reflexology. It is imperative that you explain that you do not diagnose, prescribe, or treat for a specific condition. I highly recommend a pre-printed form explaining all of this which should be signed by the client before beginning a session.

HOW MUCH PRESSURE DO YOU USE?

Naturally, the pressure used will vary with each pair of feet. The more sensitive the individual, the lighter the pressure. One sure way to check the right pressure is to watch the client's face to see if you are causing any discomfort. A note to the beginning Reflexologist: you will develop a sense of *feel* as you work and you will soon learn that some discomfort may be experienced by the client. The trained Reflexologist soon learns to distinguish between real discomfort and a *good hurt*. Divergent as that statement may seem, you will learn that one of the high points in a session is when you reach that level where your client tells you that *"it hurts, but it feels so good"*

HOW MUCH TIME IS SPENT ON EACH FOOT?

The best way to approach this is to divide your time into sections. . .ten minutes per segment. That's ten minutes per foot and then the last 20 minutes should be devoted to those systems which most need to be worked.

HOW MANY SESSIONS PER WEEK?

For optimum results, I recommend a minimum of two sessions per week for several weeks and then gradually reduce the number per week. Of course, the more chronic the problem, the longer Reflexology must be used.

But always remember, one does not have to be sick to enjoy the benefits of Reflexology. It is used as a *toner upper* by many people. To others, it is employed as a preventive, a holistic approach to health. In these cases, I recommend a session once a month, or even once every two weeks. This will depend on what it takes to maintain homeostasis for the individual.

WHAT FOOT SHOULD YOU START ON?

As my Aunt Eunice found out so many years ago, it really doesn't make any difference. I have always started on the right foot using the right hand. My recommendation is to start with that foot with which you are most comfortable. After a while, it will become almost automatic with you.

It should be noted that these holding and working positions may vary slightly for several reasons . . . the size of the foot or the worker's hands . . . this is particularly true when working with children's feet.

Now, let me finish this section by perhaps repeating myself. But it is important to you to always remember that Reflexology is an adjunctive to the health field, the same as other modalities. **We do not practice medicine.** Often when in a session and you come upon a tender spot, your client might ask you what that represents or what does that spot mean healthwise. Your best answer to that is that it simply represents a region of the body. Example of a region: a.) Head region, b.) Chest region, c.) Midsection, d.) Pelvic region. You cannot tell them that it represents a specific organ or gland. Since so many organs and glands overlap, you might be wrong in your answer anyway. You are helping nature to normalize. Tenderness indicates congestion and we are simply trying to work that out with a series of sessions, but we must always realize that there are exceptions to this . . . some people are more sensitive, some are ticklish. And the opposite is often true. They may have no tender spots and still have ill health. Often, certain medications tend to anesthetize reflexes, poor circulation and a high threshold of pain also often negate reflexes. On a heavy foot, the reflexes are sometimes deeper and will require more precise heavy pressure. Sometimes it will take two or three sessions to bring about the sensitivity. When a person is very ill, you should work for a short period of time, very lightly and more often.

REMEMBER: If you overwork the client he may have a reaction. A reaction might be uncomfortable but it is not harmful as it is nature's way of carrying away toxins.

There are many ramifications to this science of Reflexology. If you follow the rules and the training, making sure you are always aware that *you are not taking the place of the physician*, you will succeed. Reflexology is a supplement to the health field.

Chapter 15

HAND REFLEXOLOGY

"So they strengthened their hands for this good work"

Nehemiah 2:18

HAND REFLEXOLOGY

There seems to be an increasing interest today in the use of Reflexology on the hands themselves. This is an interesting evolution of interest but one with some ramifications. In my many years of experience with my Aunt, Eunice Ingham, and with the experiences of colleagues, we have found that there are basic differences when working the hands.

My own recommendation on this subject on Hand Reflexology is that the hands should be reserved for self-help. By this I mean that the hands are an excellent place to work on yourself if you can't work on your own feet or get someone else to work on them. You can work on them every day if you wish. Also your clients can easily reinforce your own work upon their feet by working the hands at their own leisure and at home between sessions. You will have to instruct them *how and where* to work their hands for *homework*.

Of course in the case of an injured foot or if a foot is missing, then working the hands becomes a necessity.

There is another occasion which must be mentioned. There are times when you will meet a person who is either sensitive or a bit shy about you working on their feet. In special cases like these, the hands will once again solve the problem.

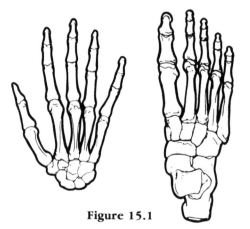

Figure 15.1

But, back to the basic differences. As you can see from the charts, it is obvious that the hand is anatomically different from the foot. (*See Figure 15.1*). The most basic is the fact that the reflexes in the hand are more compressed in the palm than those found on the sole of the foot.

Another basic deviation is that when working the hand, the holding techniques must, of necessity, be different.

When working the hand, the basic thumb technique is always used on the palm area; work the thumb up the palm, across, and at an angle in order to obtain complete coverage. And remember, when working the palms, the fingers are used for leverage on the top of the hand (I might add here that just as in most cases of working the feet, leverage is equally important when working the hands). The development of a superb technique is a necessity. (**See Figures 15.2, 15.3, 15.4**).

The index finger is primarily used on the top of the hand to work the grooves between the fingers. The thumb will be on the palm of the hand and will be used for leverage. (**See Figure 15.5**).

The fleshy "V" between the base of the thumb and the index finger is a very important reflex area. It can be worked on both the top and the bottom by the thumb as well as the fingers. This area is important simply because it represents the reflexes between the first and second zone . . . the throat, neck, and shoulder region. Work it for any associative disorder of those areas . . . whiplash, bronchitis, etc. (**See Figure 15.6**).

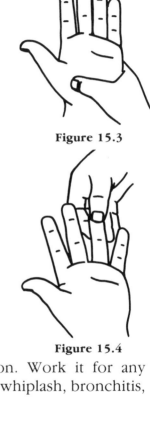

Figure 15.2

Figure 15.3

Figure 15.4

205

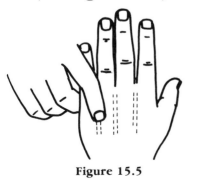

Figure 15.5

Figure 15.6

When we spoke of zone lines on the feet in *Chapter 2*, we can also apply the same to the hand. The fingers represent the zone lines as did the toes in the feet.

SOME OBSERVATIONS BASED UPON EXPERIENCE

- It is usually much easier to find tender and sore spots on the feet as compared to the hands. A natural assumption when one considers the protection afforded the feet most of the time.

- Some of the more successful results from working the hands are those reflexes associated with back problems, lymph, sinuses, whiplash. Excellent results have been obtained by working the reflexes for the neck and shoulders, breast and lungs.

- Development of an excellent working technique of the thumbs and fingers is a must when working the hands. This is an obvious necessity when you consider that the reflexes are compressed into a smaller space, they are deeper and, therefore, harder to find. The hands are not as tender as the feet so there will usually be a distinctive difference in the feeling when working on them.

- Always remember that the fingers can work the top of the hand better than the thumb. Leverage is always important when working the hand and is a fairly easy technique which can be mastered by practice.

- Don't forget the referral areas. If the foot is injured and cannot be worked, the hand may be substituted. The thumb is an excellent referral area for the great toe; the fingers can be worked for the toes. In cases of a sprained ankle, you would work the wrist.

- The hands are an excellent place to work on yourself if you can't work on your own feet or get someone else to work on them. You can work on them every day if you wish.

As in the foot, the hand orientation includes: (***See Figure 15.7***).

- The tip of the fingers
- The back of the hand
- The palm of the hand
- The heel of the hand
- The inside of the hand (medial)
- The outside of the hand (lateral)

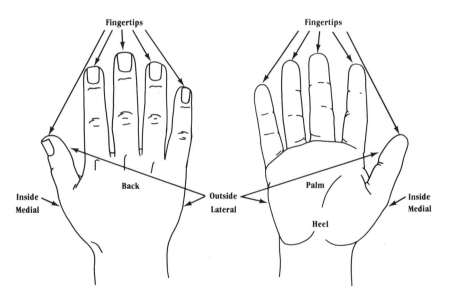

Figure 15.7

The theory is the same as for the foot . . . the right hand for the right half of the body; the left hand for the left half of the body. As with working on the foot it is very important to use the inside corner of the thumb or finger when working on the hands.

For the approximate location of the reflexes in the hands refer to the hand charts at the back of this book.

Chapter 16

INTERNATIONAL INSTITUTE
OF REFLEXOLOGY®

"There must be perfect harmony among the various parts of the body"

Galen (2nd Century Physician)

INTERNATIONAL INSTITUTE
OF REFLEXOLOGY®

The **INTERNATIONAL INSTITUTE OF REFLEXOLOGY** was formed in 1973 to carry on the great work of EUNICE INGHAM and spread the word about *"THE ORIGINAL INGHAM METHOD OF REFLEXOLOGY"* throughout the world.

The **INTERNATIONAL INSTITUTE OF REFLEXOLOGY** is headed by DWIGHT C. BYERS, Today's Leading Authority on Foot Reflexology. Mr. Byers is the Nephew of the late EUNICE INGHAM, the originator who researched and developed Reflexology as it is known today throughout the world.

The **INTERNATIONAL INSTITUTE OF REFLEXOLOGY** is the **only** organization that teaches *"THE ORIGINAL INGHAM METHOD OF REFLEXOLOGY"*. Their experienced and knowledgeable staff provide the **best** training experience possible on an INTERNATIONAL basis.

We present a concentrated, dynamic presentation on the theory and techniques. After you read this technical book you will want to attend one of our seminars and learn these techniques properly, as you cannot learn this from books alone. The seminars consist of lectures with many visual aids and you will personally apply and receive these techniques. Once you take the seminar you become a lifetime member of the **INTERNATIONAL INSTITUTE OF REFLEXOLOGY**, which entitles you to attend any future seminars, anywhere and as often as you desire. Continuing education (following instructional courses) is highly desirable. The more you attend, the better REFLEXOLOGIST you will become and the better you will maintain your skills and broaden your knowledge.

The **INTERNATIONAL INSTITUTE OF REFLEXOLOGY** also offers to its members an advanced class and CERTIFICATION PROGRAM consisting of a written and practical exam. There is also a WORLD-WIDE referral service available.

These Seminars are for everyone . . . professional and lay people alike.

If you wish to receive information regarding seminars offered in your area or related books and charts, write to:

INTERNATIONAL INSTITUTE OF REFLEXOLOGY
P. O. BOX 12642
ST. PETERSBURG, FLORIDA 33733-2642 U.S.A.
813-343-4811

SYSTEMS DISORDERS

The following pages represent a compilation of those disorders with which the practicing Reflexologist should become familiar.

The disorders and their associative reflexes are listed **only** as a guide to help you become more proficient in working these areas.

In no way is this list to be construed as, nor used for, diagnostic purposes. Diagnosis is the perogative of the physician. **Reflexologists do not diagnose nor prescribe at any time in any manner.**

D.C.B.

DISORDER	REFLEX
Acne	Liver, Adrenals, All Glands, Kidneys, Intestines, Thyroid, Diaphragm
Adenoids	Great Toes, Pituitary
Alcoholism	Liver, Pancreas, Diaphragm
Anemia	Spleen, Liver
Angina Pectoris	Heart/Lung, Cervicals, Thoracics, Sigmoid Colon, Diaphragm
Ankles (swollen)	Kidneys, Adrenals, Lymph System; Referral Area: Wrist
Appendicitis	Ileocecal, Diaphragm
Arms (Hands)	Cervicals, Upper Thoracics, Shoulder, Hip
Arteriosclerosis	All Glands; work entire foot
Arthritis	Entire Foot; Work Reflex to Affected Area
Asthma	Chest/Lung, Adrenals, Ileocecal, Diaphragm

DISORDER	REFLEX
Atherosclerosis	Thyroid, All Glands; Work Entire Foot
Bed Wetting	Kidneys, Diaphragm, Ureters, Adrenals, Lower Spice
Bell's Palsy	Cervicals, Diaphragm
Bladder Problems	Bladder, Kidneys, Ureters, Adrenals, Lower Spine
Breasts (lumps)	Chest/Lung, Lymph System, Pituitary
Bright's Disease	Kidneys
Bronchitis	Chest/Lung, Ileocecal, Diaphragm, Adrenals
Bunion	Work around and directly on Bunion
Bursitis	Reflex to Affected Area, Adrenals, Referral Area to Affected Area
Calluses, Corns	Around and directly on them
Cataracts	Eye Reflex, Neck Area, Cervicals, All Toes, Pituitary, Kidneys
Chest Pains	Sigmoid, Diaphragm, Chest/Lung
Childhood Diseases	All Glands, Diaphragm
Cholesterol	Thyroid, Liver
Cirrhosis of the Liver	Liver, Pancreas, All Glands
Coccyx (Lower Backache)	Whole Spine, Kidney, Hip, Shoulder
Colds	Chest/Lung, Adrenals, Intestines, Pituitary, Lymph System, All Toes
Colitis	Colon, Liver, Adrenal, Lower Spine, Diaphragm, Gall Bladder
Conjunctivitis	Eye Reflex, All Toes, Neck, Kidneys
Constipation	Liver, Gall Bladder, Diaphragm, Adrenals, Lower Spine, Ileocecal, Sigmoid
Cramps (feet, legs, etc.)	Hip/Knee, Hip/Sciatic, Lower Spine, Parathyroid, Adrenals

DISORDER	REFLEX
Cramps (menstrual)	Uterus, Ovaries, Fallopian Tubes, Diaphragm, Lower Spine, All Glands
Croup	Diaphragm, Bronchials, Chest/Lung, Ileocecal, All Toes
Cystitis	Kidneys, Bladder, Ureter Tubes, Lower Spine, Adrenals
Deafness	Ear Reflex, Cervicals, Side of Neck, Great Toes
Diabetes	Pancreas, Liver, All Glands
Diarrhea	Ascending Colon, Transverse Colon, Diaphragm, Liver, Adrenals
Diverticulitis	Colon, Diaphragm, Adrenals, Lower Spine, Liver, Gall Bladder
Dizziness	Side of Neck, Ear Reflex, Cervicals
Drug Addiction	All Glands, Diaphragm, Liver, Kidneys
Dry Skin	Thyroid, Adrenals
Ears	Ear Reflex, All Toes, Throat/Neck (Eustachian Tube)
Eczema	Diaphragm, Liver, Kidneys, Intestines, Adrenals, All Glands, Thyroid
Edema	Lymph System, Kidneys, Adrenals
Emphysema	Ileocecal, Adrenals, Chest/Lung, Lymph System, Diaphragm
Encephalitis	Great Toe, All Toes, All Glands
Epilepsy	Diaphragm, Colon, Ileocecal, Whole Spine, Neck Area, All Glands
Eye Conditions	Eye Reflex, Throat/Neck, All Toes, Kidneys, Cervicals
Fainting	Pituitary
Fatigue (General)	Adrenals, Diaphragm, All Glands, Whole Spine

DISORDER	REFLEX
Feet (cold and sweaty)	Liver, Intestines, Kidney, All Glands
Fever	Pituitary
Flatulance	Intestines, Stomach, Liver, Gall Bladder, Pancreas
Fluid Retention (edema)	Lymph System, Kidneys, Adrenals
Fracture	Reflex to affected area on foot, also Referral Area
Gall Stones	Liver, Gall Bladder, Thyroid
Gas Pains	Stomach, Diaphragm, Intestines, Liver
Glaucoma	Eye Reflex, Throat/Neck, All Toes, Kidneys, Cervicals
Gout	Kidneys, Reflex to affected area
Growths (abnormal)	Pituitary, Reflex to affected area
Hay Fever	Ileocecal, All Toes, Colon, All Glands, Chest/Lung
Halitosis	Stomach, Liver, Intestines, Great Toes
Headache (General)	Whole Spine, Diaphragm, All Glands, All toes
Heartburn	Diaphragm, Gall Bladder, Pancreas, Stomach, All Glands
Heart Conditions	Chest/Lung, Diaphragm, Cervicals, Sigmoid, Thoracics
Hemorrhoids	Diaphragm, Adrenals, Rectum, Sigmoid, Lower Spine; also Chronic area up the back of the heel
Hernia (abdominal)	Groin Area, Colon, Adrenals
Hiatus Hernia	Diaphragm, Stomach, Adrenals
Hiccoughs	Diaphragm, Stomach
High Blood Pressure (Hypertension)	Diaphragm; and also Kidneys, Pituitary, Adrenals, Thyroid

DISORDER	REFLEX
High Cholesterol Level	Thyroid, Liver
Hip	Hip/Sciatic, Hip/Knee, Lower Spine, Shoulder
Hot Flashes	Diaphragm, All Glands, Reproductive System, Chronic Uterus Area
Hyperactivity	Diaphragm, All Glands
Hypoglycemia	Pancreas, All Glands, Liver
Hysterectomy	Adrenals, Thyroid, Pituitary, Uterus, Ovaries, Fallopian Tubes, Diaphragm, Chronic Uterus Area
Impotence	Reproductive System, All Glands, Whole Spine, Diaphragm
Incontinence	Ureters, Bladder, Kidneys, Adrenals, Lower Spine
Indigestion	Liver, Gall Bladder, Stomach, Intestines, Diaphragm
Infections	Adrenals, Lymph System, Region or area affected
Infertility	Reproductive System, All Glands, Whole Spine, Diaphragm
Influenza	Chest/Lung, Diaphragm, Intestines, All Glands, Lymph System
Insomnia	Diaphragm, All Glands
Jaundice	Liver
Kidney Stones	Ureter Tubes, Kidneys, Bladder, Diaphragm, Parathyroid
Knees	Hip/Knee, Hip/Sciatic, Lower Spine; Referral Area: Elbow
Laryngitis	Throat, Chest/Lung, Diaphragm, Lymph System, All Toes
Legs (swelling)	Lymph System, Kidneys, Adrenals

DISORDER	REFLEX
Leukemia	All Glands, Lymph System, Spleen
Liver Conditions	Liver, Gall Bladder, Whole Spine
Low Blood Pressure (Hypotension)	Adrenals; and also Pituitary, Thyroid
Lupus	All Glands, Intestines, Liver, Whole Spine
Meningitis	Great Toes, Whole Spine, All Glands
Menopause (hot flashes)	Diaphragm, All Glands, Reproductive System, Chronic Uterus Area
Menstrual Cramps	Uterus, Ovaries, Fallopian Tubes, Lower Spine, All Glands, Diaphragm
Migraine	Whole Spine, Diaphragm, Pituitary, Great Toes, Intestines
Morning Sickness	All Glands, Diaphragm, Stomach
Motion Sickness (Land, Sea, Air)	Ear Reflex, Diaphragm, Neck, Spine
Mucus (Sinus)	Ileocecal, Chest/Lung, All Toes, Adrenals
Multiple Sclerosis	Whole Spine, All Glands, Diaphragm
Nausea	Liver, Gall Bladder, Stomach, Diaphragm
Neck Tension	Neck, Cervicals, Shoulders
Nephritis	Kidneys
Nervousness	Diaphragm, All Glands, Whole Spine
Neuritis	Spine, Diaphragm, Glands, Corresponding Reflex Area
Ovaries (Ovarian Cysts)	Ovaries, Pituitary, All Glands, Uterus, Fallopian Tubes
Paralysis	Whole Spine, Brain, Related Reflex Area
Parkinson's Disease	Whole Spine, All Glands, Diaphragm, Chest/Lung
Perspiring Hands and Feet	All Glands, Liver, Intestines, Kidneys, Diaphragm

DISORDER	REFLEX
Phlebitis	Adrenals, Colon, Liver; Referral Area: Arm
Pink Eye (conjunctivitis)	Eye Reflex, All Toes, Neck, Kidneys
Pleurisy	Lymph System, Adrenals, Diaphragm, Chest/Lung
Pneumonia	Chest/Lung, Diaphragm, Intestines, All Glands, Lymph System
Pregnancy	All Glands, Whole Spine, Reproductive System, Bladder, Diaphragm
Prostate	Reproductive Glands, Bladder, Lower Spine, Pituitary, Adrenals, Chronic Prostate Area
Psoriasis	Thyroid, Adrenals, Liver, Diaphragm, Kidneys, Intestines, All Glands
Pyorrhea	Great Toes, All Glands
Ruptured Disk	Work affected Areas of Spine
Sciatica	Hip/Sciatic, Hip/Knee, Lower Spine, Shoulder, Chronic Sciatic Area
Scoliosis	Whole Spine, All Glands, Chest/Lung, Shoulder
Shingles	Diaphragm, All Glands, Whole Spine
Shoulders	Shoulder (top and bottom), Cervicals, Hip, Neck
Sinusitis	All Toes, Ileocecal, Adrenals, Chest/Lung
Smell	Great Toes, All Toes
Sore Throat	Lymph System, All Toes, Great Toes, Adrenals, Cervicals
Sprain or Strain	Work Reflex Area on Foot, Referral Area to affected Area
Spur on Heel	All around Spur and directly on Spur

219

DISORDER	REFLEX
Stroke	Tip of Great Toe (opposite side from paralysis), Other Toes, Reflexes to affected Areas
Sty	Eye Reflex, Neck Area, All Toes
Swelling (Edema)	Lymph System, Kidneys, Adrenals
Taste	All Toes, Middle ⅓ of Great Toes
Teeth and Gums	All Toes, Middle ⅓ of Great Toes
Tension (Nervous)	Diaphragm, All Glands, Whole Spine
Thyroid	Pituitary, Adrenal, Thyroid
Tic douloureux	Neck, Cervicals, Diaphragm
Tinnitis	Ear Reflex, Cervicals, Neck, Small Toes
Tonsillitis	Great Toes, Lymph System, All Toes, Adrenals, Cervicals
Toothache	All Toes, Middle ⅓ of Great Toes
Tremors	Whole Spine, Diaphragm
Tumors	Pituitary, All Glands, Reflex Pertaining to Location of Tumor
Ulcers	Diaphragm, Stomach, Duodenum, Reflex pertaining to Location of Ulcer
Urinary Trouble	Ureter Tubes, Bladder, Kidneys, Adrenals, Lower Spine
Varicose Veins	Colon, Liver, Adrenals, Referral Area: Arm
Vertigo	Ear Reflex, Neck, Cervicals, Great Toes
Vitality (Low)	Adrenals, Diaphragm, All Glands, Whole Spine
Whiplash	Top and Bottom of Foot Between Great Toe and Second Toe, Whole Spine, 7th Cervical
Wrist (Sprain or Break)	Referral Area: Ankle

A CONCLUDING THOUGHT
from
"Stories The Feet Can Tell"

Let me remind you that Reflexology is a means of equalizing the circulation. We all know circulation is life. Stagnation is death. Everything around us that is alive is in motion.

Everything in the universe is governed by the law of motion, which is one of God's great infallible laws of nature. It is from the earth, sun, and water which are constantly in motion that we receive our creative forces which are followed by growth, maturity and decay. Nothing stands still. Our vitality is either increasing or decreasing according to the quality and circulation of our bloodstream.

Study for a moment the life of a sturdy oak, which from a tiny acorn grows. Stop and observe how it lifts its leafy arms toward Heaven to receive from the passing breezes the exercise necessary to strengthen its root supply, increasing the capacity to gather moisture and nourishment necessary to furnish and keep the sap flowing freely through every part. If we cut off the roots sufficiently to rob it of its life-giving sap, how long will the tree be green and full of life?

In the face of this shall we forget the necessity of keeping our whole body in motion; every part in perfect rhythm.

It is my sincere wish that this technique of Foot and Hand Reflexology will stand side by side with other great therapy works in the onward march of science and progress.

221

EUNICE D. INGHAM

1938

INDEX

Reflexology

HAND CHARTS

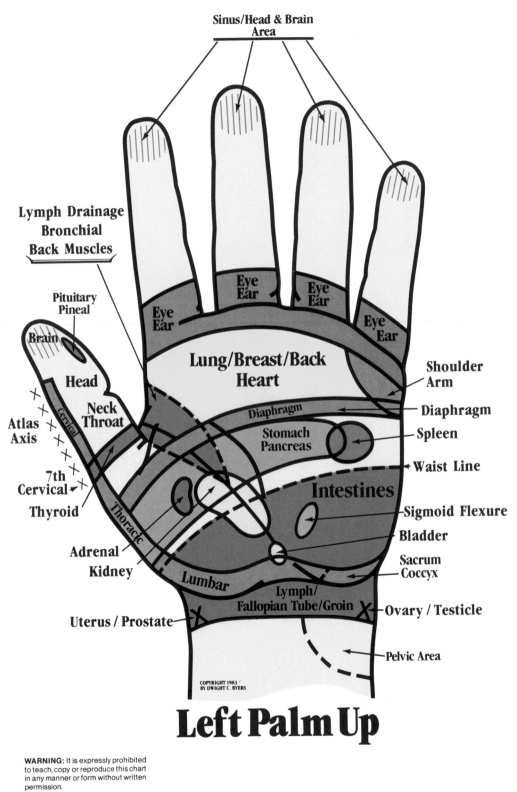

Left Palm Up

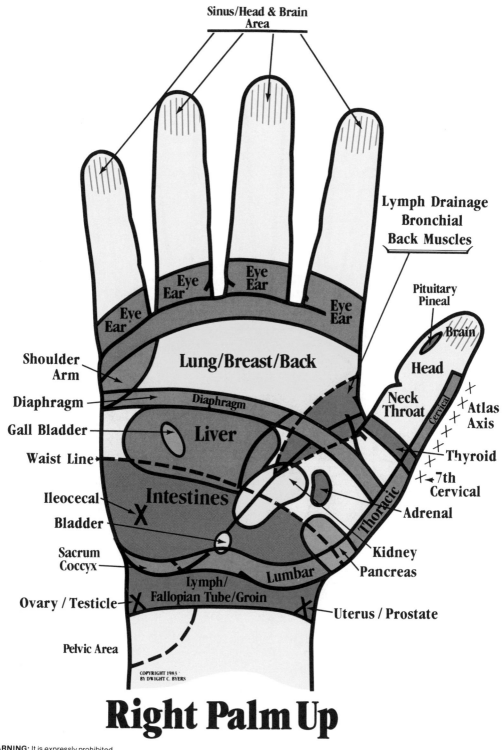

Sinus/Head & Brain Area

Lymph Drainage
Bronchial
Back Muscles

Eye Ear

Eye Ear

Eye Ear

Pituitary Pineal

Brain

Head

Shoulder Arm

Lung/Breast/Back

Neck Throat

Cervical

Atlas Axis

Diaphragm

Diaphragm

Gall Bladder

Liver

Thyroid

Waist Line

7th Cervical

Ileocecal

Intestines

Thoracic

Adrenal

Bladder

Sacrum Coccyx

Lumbar

Kidney

Pancreas

Ovary / Testicle

Lymph/ Fallopian Tube/Groin

Uterus / Prostate

Pelvic Area

COPYRIGHT 1983
BY DWIGHT C. BYERS

Right Palm Up

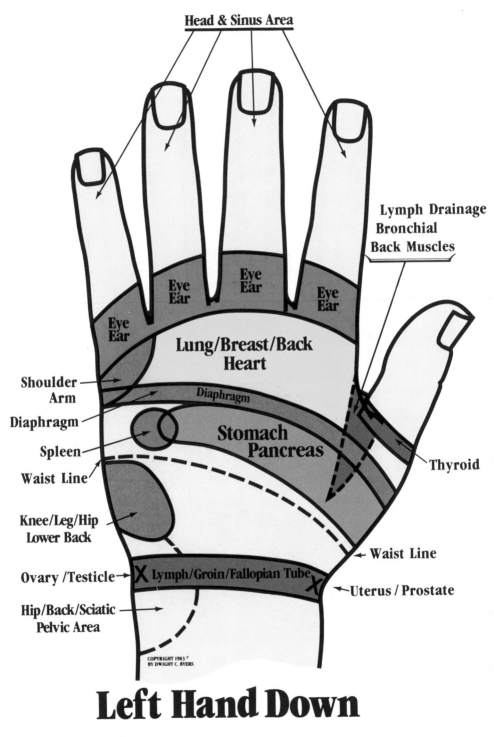

Head & Sinus Area

Lymph Drainage
Bronchial
Back Muscles

Eye
Ear

Eye
Ear

Eye
Ear

Eye
Ear

Lung/Breast/Back
Heart

Shoulder
Arm

Diaphragm

Diaphragm

Spleen

Stomach
Pancreas

Waist Line

Thyroid

Knee/Leg/Hip
Lower Back

Waist Line

Ovary /Testicle

X Lymph/Groin/Fallopian Tube X

Uterus / Prostate

Hip/Back/Sciatic
Pelvic Area

COPYRIGHT 1983 ©
BY DWIGHT C. BYERS

Left Hand Down

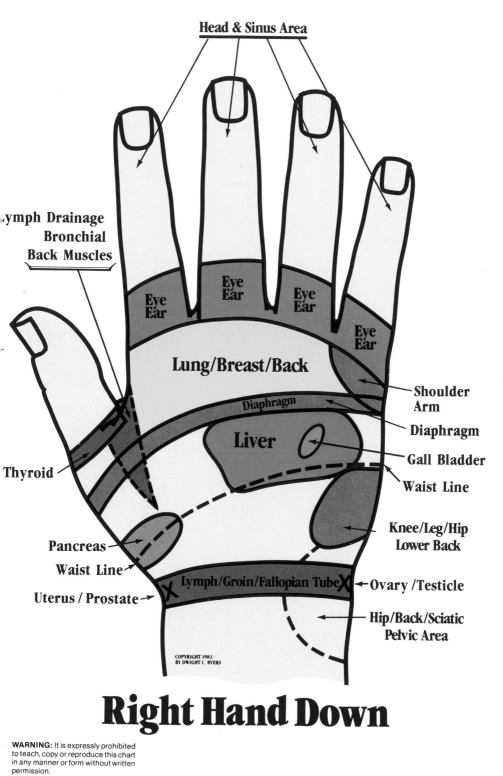

Head & Sinus Area

Lymph Drainage
Bronchial
Back Muscles

Eye Ear

Eye Ear

Eye Ear

Eye Ear

Lung/Breast/Back

Shoulder Arm

Diaphragm

Diaphragm

Liver

Gall Bladder

Waist Line

Thyroid

Knee/Leg/Hip
Lower Back

Pancreas

Waist Line

Uterus / Prostate

X Lymph/Groin/Fallopian Tube X

Ovary /Testicle

Hip/Back/Sciatic
Pelvic Area

COPYRIGHT 1983
BY DWIGHT C. BYERS

Right Hand Down

Reflexology

FOOT CHART

PULL OUT CHART ➔